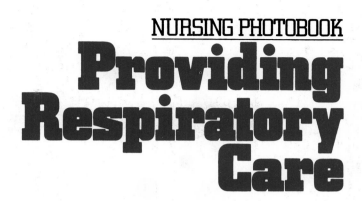

NURSING PHOTOBOOK
Providing Respiratory Care

NURSING80 PHOTOBOOKS
INTERMED COMMUNICATIONS, INC.
HORSHAM, PENNSYLVANIA

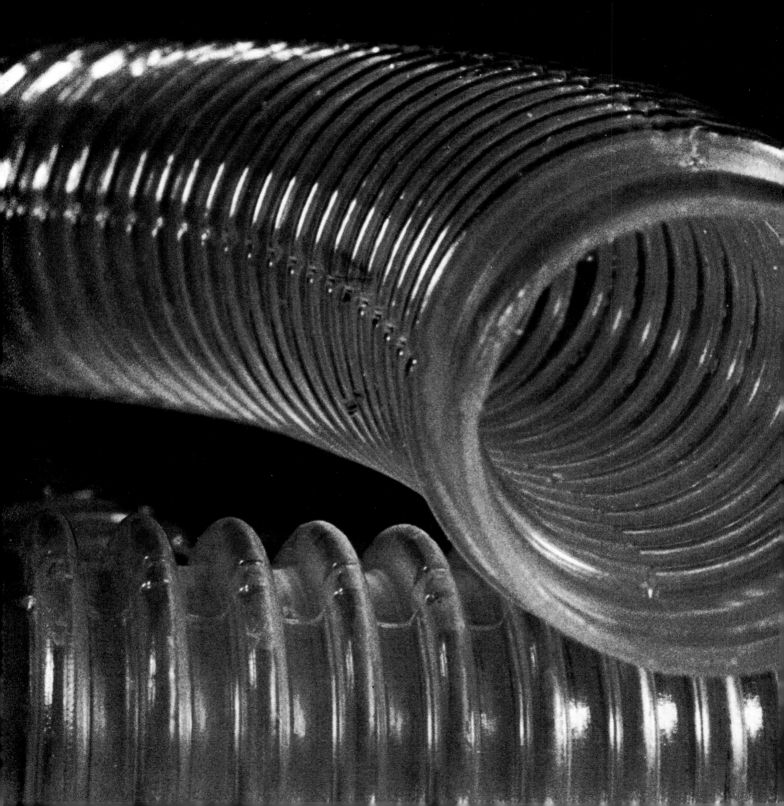

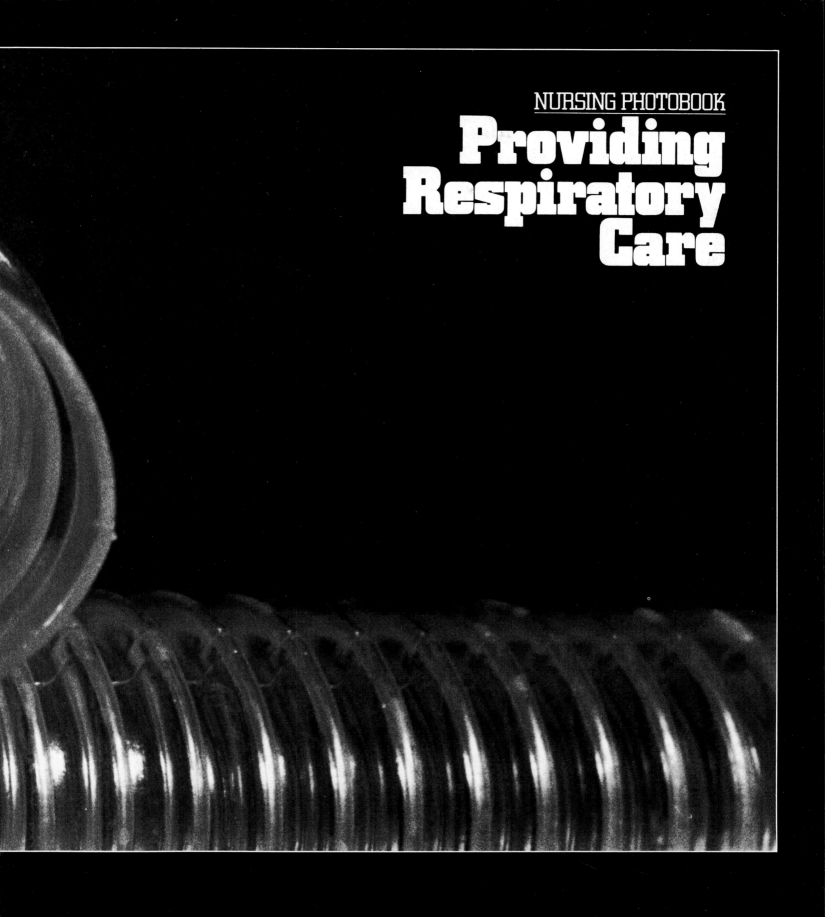

Providing Respiratory Care

Nursing80®
Photobook™ **Series**
PUBLISHER
Eugene W. Jackson

EDITORIAL DIRECTOR
Jean Robinson

CLINICAL DIRECTOR
Barbara McVan, RN

ART DIRECTOR
Burton P. Pollack

MANUFACTURING DIRECTOR
Bernard Haas

**Intermed Communications
Book Division**
PUBLISHER
Daniel L. Cheney

DIRECTOR, GRAPHICS
John C. Isely

DIRECTOR, RESEARCH
Elizabeth O'Brien

DIRECTOR, PURCHASING
Wilhelm R. Saake

Staff for this volume
BOOK EDITORS
Sanford Robinson
Patricia Russo

CLINICAL EDITOR
Helene Ritting Nawrocki, RN

ASSOCIATE CLINICAL EDITORS
Theresa Croushore, RN
Mary Gyetvan, RN, BSEd.

ASSOCIATE EDITORS
Katherine W. Carey
Roger Schiffman
Richard Samuel West

COPY EDITORS
Pat Hamilton
Barbara Hodgson

EDITORIAL ASSISTANTS
Margaret Andrews
Evelyn M. James

PHOTOGRAPHER
Paul A. Cohen

DESIGNERS
Lisa A. Gilde
Linda A. Jovinelly

PHOTOGRAPHER'S ASSISTANT
Thomas Staudenmayer

ART PRODUCTION MANAGER
Wilbur D. Davidson

ART COORDINATOR
Gloria Moyer

ART ASSISTANTS
Lorraine Carbo
Diane Fox
Robert Perry
Robert H. Renn
Edward Rosanio
Sandra Simms

RESEARCHER AND INDEXER
Vonda Heller

TYPOGRAPHY MANAGER
David C. Kosten

TYPOGRAPHY ASSISTANTS
Diane Paluba
Thomas E. Roch

PRODUCTION MANAGER
Robert L. Dean, Jr.

PRODUCTION ASSISTANT
Doreen K. Stowers

ILLUSTRATORS
Jean Gardner
Tom Herbert
Robert Jackson
John R. Murphy
Bud Yingling

**Clinical consultants
for this volume**
Margaret Fuhs, RN, MSN,
Pulmonary Clinical Specialist,
Hospital of the University of
Pennsylvania, Philadelphia.

Victoria J. Nimon, RN,
Charge Nurse ICU,
Winter Park Memorial Hospital,
Winter Park, Florida.

Cover photo
Seymour Mednick

Library of Congress Cataloging in Publication Data

Main entry under title:

Providing respiratory care.

(Nursing Photobook)
Bibliography: p.
Includes index.
   1. Respiratory disease nursing. [DNLM:
1. Respiratory tract diseases. WY163 P969]
RC735.5.P76   610.73'6   79-21639
ISBN 0-916730-17-4

Contents

Contributors

Barbara Clippinger received her RN from Temple University, Philadelphia, Pennsylvania. She is a staff nurse in the head and neck tumor clinic at Temple University Hospital, Philadelphia. Ms. Clippinger is a member of the Society of Otorhinolaryngology and Head and Neck Nurses, and the American Cancer Society.

Shirley L. Egger is a clinical instructor of intensive care nursing at Toronto Western Hospital, Canada. She graduated from St. Joseph's School of Nursing, Hamilton, Ontario, Canada.

Margaret Fuhs, one of the advisors on this book, is a pulmonary clinical specialist at the Hospital of the University of Pennsylvania in Philadelphia. She received her BSN from the Columbia University School of Nursing, and her MSN from the University of Pennsylvania. Ms. Fuhs is a doctoral candidate in nursing at Catholic University of America, Washington, D.C.

Frances J. Lekwart received her BSN from Houston Baptist University and her MSN from the University of California at San Francisco. She is a respiratory clinical specialist at Jefferson Davis Hospital, Houston, Texas. Ms. Lekwart is a member of the Texas Nurses' Association, American Nurses' Association, and the American Association of Critical Care Nurses.

Shirley Marshburn is a graduate of St. Margaret's Hospital School of Nursing, Montgomery, Alabama, and is a BSN candidate at Southern Missionary College, Orlando, Florida. She is a supervisor in the emergency department at Winter Park Memorial Hospital, Florida. Ms. Marshburn is a member of the Emergency Department Nurses' Association, and the Southeastern Hospital Conference Education Committee.

Victoria J. Nimon, also an advisor on this book, is a charge nurse in the intensive care unit at Winter Park Memorial Hospital in Florida. A graduate of St. Joseph's School of Practical Nursing, Ms. Nimon received her AS in nursing from Valencia Community College, Orlando, Florida. She is a member of the American Heart Association.

Jan Stephen Tecklin is a physical therapist and instructor in the cystic fibrosis/pediatric pulmonary center, Department of Pediatrics, Hahnemann Medical College and Hospital, Philadelphia. He received his BS in health and physical education from West Chester State College in Pennsylvania, and his physical therapy certification from the University of Pennsylvania, Philadelphia. He is a member of the American Physical Therapy Association, and the American Thoracic Society.

Bruce Paul Toben received his AS in Respiratory Therapy Technology from the Community College of Philadelphia, Pennsylvania. He is the chief of respiratory therapy services at Germantown Dispensary and Hospital, Philadelphia. Also, Mr. Toben is an instructor in accelerated respiratory therapy technology for the community services division of Community College of Philadelphia. He is a member of the American Association for Respiratory Therapy, American Lung Association, and American Association of Physicians Assistants.

Johnsie Whitt Woody is a graduate of Petersburg General Hospital School of Nursing, Virginia. She is a respiratory nurse clinician at Duke University Hospital, Durham, North Carolina. Ms. Woody is a member of the Board of Directors of the North Carolina Lung Association.

Introduction

What do you need to know about respiratory care? More than an ordinary textbook can tell you—or even your hospital's procedure manual. A textbook long on theory may short-change you on vital how-to instructions. And your hospital's procedure manual won't provide more than written basics.

But count yourself fortunate. The publishers of *Nursing80* have come to your rescue. This NURSING PHOTOBOOK goes beyond what you've encountered in textbooks and manuals; it puts you right in the picture. Everything you need to know is explained *visually* in photos and illustrations. You no longer have to *wonder* how certain steps in a procedure are done, because this PHOTOBOOK will *show* you.

For example, you'll see how to reposition and tape an oral endotracheal tube; how to accomplish emergency trach tube reinsertion; and how to teach home trach care. You'll see how to draw blood from a radial artery, use a venturi mask, and give humidified oxygen to a patient with a tracheostomy.

If you're confused about ventilators, this PHOTOBOOK will acquaint you with the more common ones. It'll also show you how to troubleshoot ventilator problems and manage the ventilated patient.

The last section of this PHOTOBOOK illustrates chest tube management, including many procedures you may be unfamiliar with: for example, how to set up an Emerson pump, cope with two- and three-bottle drainage systems, and deal with chest tube emergencies.

We're aware that procedures and views on many controversial aspects of respiratory care can vary from hospital to hospital, and that some procedures illustrated in this PHOTOBOOK require special training you may not have had. But that's what good nursing is all about. Improving your skills and keeping up with the latest techniques. To this end, we've enlisted the help and expertise of contributors from all around the United States and Canada.

And these contributors have come up with the *extras* you expect from us: nursing tips, timesavers, insights, and improvisations. Plus those valuable warnings about pitfalls that'll help you avoid errors and accidents. You'll learn to do respiratory care procedures *correctly,* because you learn from the *working experts.* No better way exists for you to gain the confidence you need and increase your efficiency.

Our goal? We at NURSING PHOTOBOOKS want to help you become a better nurse. Why? Because we know you'll use your increased skills and knowledge to help your patients.

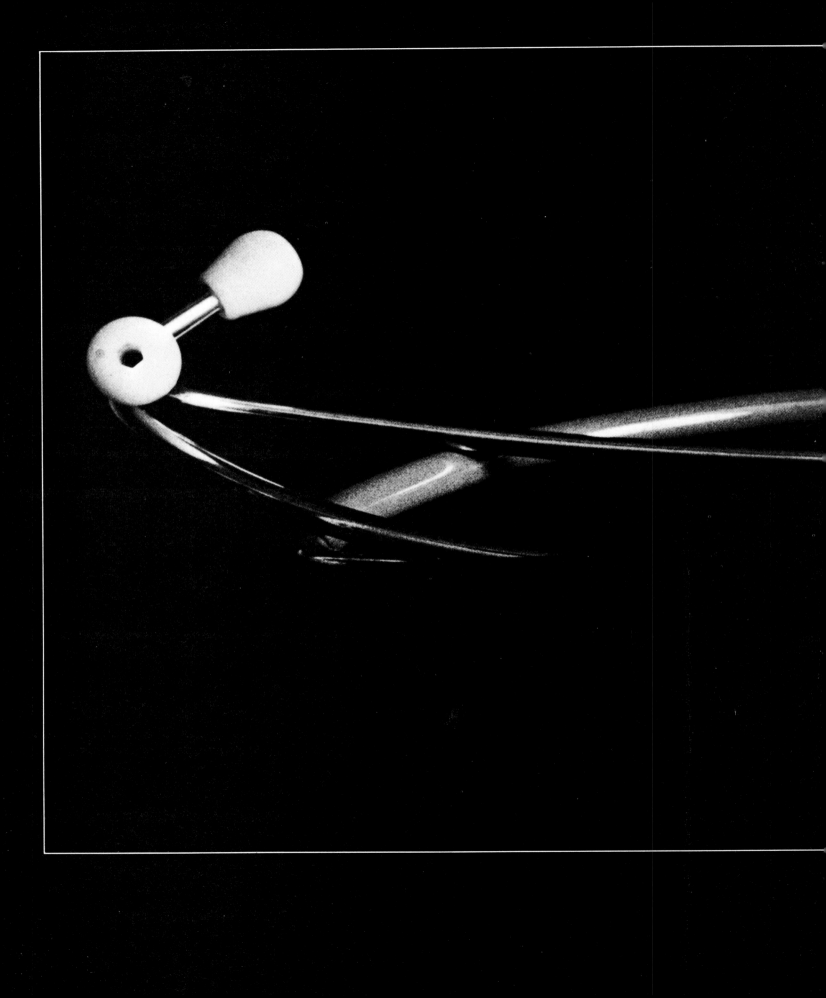

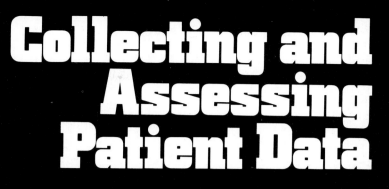

Collecting and Assessing Patient Data

Respiratory basics
Chest assessment
Respiratory patterns
Respiratory sounds

Respiratory basics

Suppose you're interviewing and assessing a patient with a respiratory problem. How well you understand respiratory anatomy and function will affect your evaluation. Knowing what to ask your patient— and what his answers may indicate—are also important. If you're uncertain, you'll have trouble making an accurate assessment. To help, we've illustrated the respiratory system anatomy on these pages, so you can review the basics you learned in school. We've also included questions to ask your patient in your initial interview.

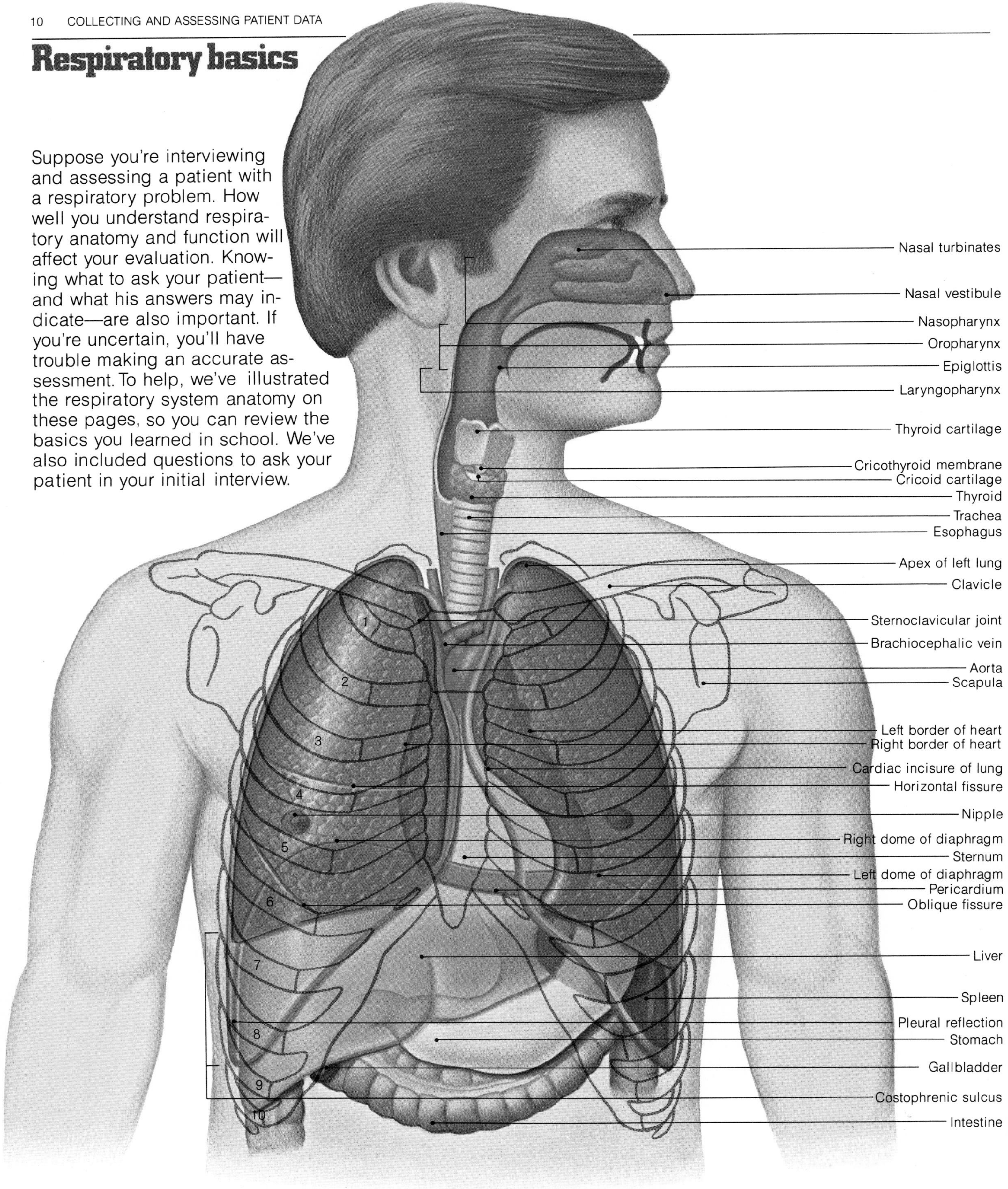

Nasal turbinates
Nasal vestibule
Nasopharynx
Oropharynx
Epiglottis
Laryngopharynx
Thyroid cartilage
Cricothyroid membrane
Cricoid cartilage
Thyroid
Trachea
Esophagus
Apex of left lung
Clavicle
Sternoclavicular joint
Brachiocephalic vein
Aorta
Scapula
Left border of heart
Right border of heart
Cardiac incisure of lung
Horizontal fissure
Nipple
Right dome of diaphragm
Sternum
Left dome of diaphragm
Pericardium
Oblique fissure
Liver
Spleen
Pleural reflection
Stomach
Gallbladder
Costophrenic sulcus
Intestine

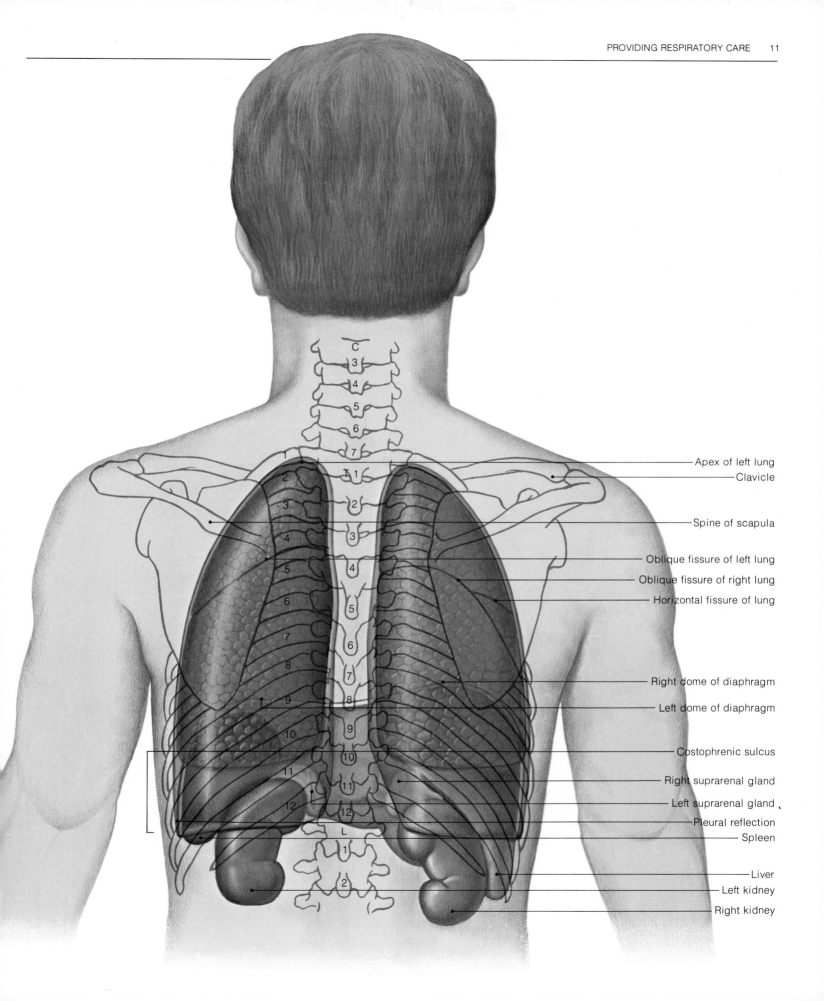

Apex of left lung

Clavicle

Spine of scapula

Oblique fissure of left lung

Oblique fissure of right lung

Horizontal fissure of lung

Right dome of diaphragm

Left dome of diaphragm

Costophrenic sulcus

Right suprarenal gland

Left suprarenal gland

Pleural reflection

Spleen

Liver

Left kidney

Right kidney

Respiratory basics

The illustrations will help you visualize the respiratory system and understand how gases are exchanged between alveolar air and capillary blood.

For a close-up look at one part of the lungs' alveolar capillary network, study the simplified, stylized diagram below. Follow the pulmonary artery, with its supply of mixed venous blood. When it reaches the lungs, its terminal branches enter the alveolar capillary network shown in the middle of the diagram. It's here that oxygen and carbon dioxide are exchanged.

During the gas exchange process, oxygen and carbon dioxide continually diffuse across a very thin pulmonary membrane. To understand the direction in which they move, remember that gases move from areas of higher pressure to areas of lower pressure. If you study the pressures on the diagram, you can see how carbon dioxide diffuses from the venous end of the capillary into the alveolus, and oxygen diffuses from the alveolus into the capillary.

This oxygenated blood then flows into a pulmonary vein branch. From there, it's carried throughout the body so it can deliver oxygen to body cells.

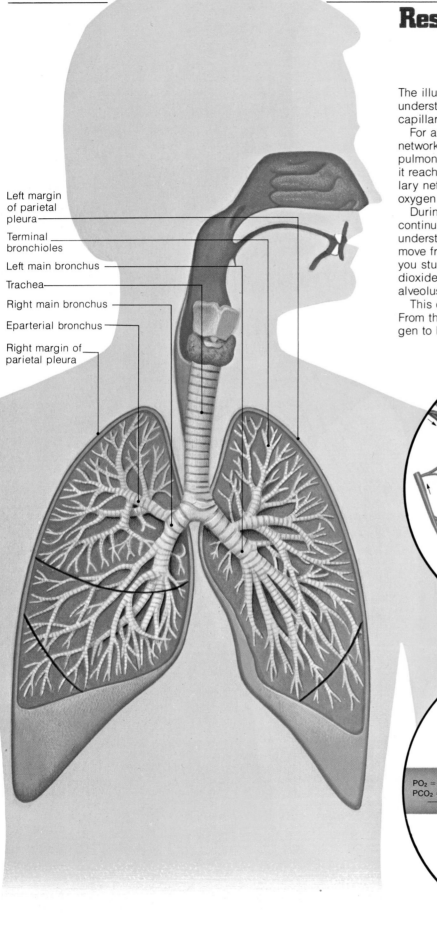

Left margin of parietal pleura

Terminal bronchioles

Left main bronchus

Trachea

Right main bronchus

Eparterial bronchus

Right margin of parietal pleura

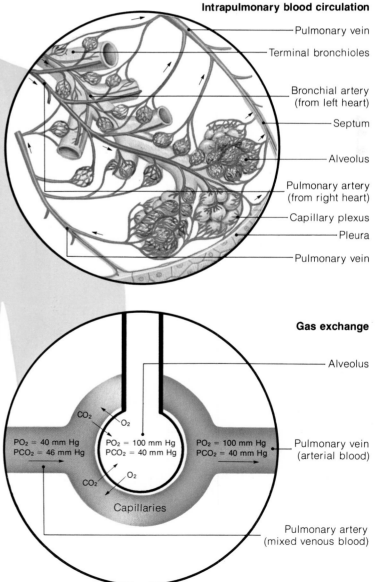

Intrapulmonary blood circulation

Pulmonary vein

Terminal bronchioles

Bronchial artery (from left heart)

Septum

Alveolus

Pulmonary artery (from right heart)

Capillary plexus

Pleura

Pulmonary vein

Gas exchange

Alveolus

$PO_2 = 40$ mm Hg
$PCO_2 = 46$ mm Hg

$PO_2 = 100$ mm Hg
$PCO_2 = 40$ mm Hg

$PO_2 = 100$ mm Hg
$PCO_2 = 40$ mm Hg

CO_2 O_2

CO_2 O_2

Capillaries

Pulmonary vein (arterial blood)

Pulmonary artery (mixed venous blood)

Chest assessment

Is your patient having trouble breathing?
How can you tell if your patient needs help to breathe more easily? Observe him closely, and ask yourself these questions:
- Is his breathing noisy and labored?
- Does his abdomen protrude with each breath?
- Is he using the accessory muscles in his neck to breathe?
- Are his nostrils dilated or flared?
- Does he have a fearful, anxious look?
- Does he clutch or grasp at his gown and bed linen?

- Does he seem confused or unusually restless?
- Is his skin cool to the touch?
- Do his fingernail beds, earlobes, and mouth mucosa (particularly under the tongue) look cyanotic? *Note:* If your patient has dark skin, also check his conjunctiva, palms of hands, and soles of feet.
- Does a vital-sign check show an increase in respirations, blood pressure, and heart rate?

All these signs indicate that your patient's having trouble breathing. Take steps immediately to ease his distress.

Interviewing your patient: What to ask

Does your new patient have a respiratory problem? Use these guidelines to help you focus your initial interview on his problem and its symptoms. Carefully document his answers in your nurses' notes.

Begin by asking your patient general questions that require more than a monosyllabic response; for example:

- When did you first notice the symptoms?

- What were you doing when they occurred?

- Are those symptoms better or worse now? What seems to make them better or worse?

- What medication, if any, have you taken to relieve them? Does it seem to help? (Always try to find out if the patient's taking antibiotics, digitalis, bronchodilators, diuretics, or steroids. If he's on steroids, he'll need to continue taking them in the hospital.)

- Do you use any breathing aids at home? For example, oxygen, IPPB, a nebulizer or humidifier? (If he does, he may need them in the hospital.)

Next, concentrate on specific symptoms. If he complains of dyspnea, ask:

- Does your feeling of breathlessness occur when you rest? Lie flat? Walk on level ground? Up a flight of steps? During normal activity? When you're under tension?

- How far can you walk before you feel breathless? What symptom makes you stop walking? For example, does your heart pound? Or do your legs feel weak?

- How long have you had this symptom? Is it better or worse now than before?

If he complains of cough, ask:

- Do you cough when you wake up, during the day, at night, in bad weather? Do you bring up phlegm? What consistency? Do you have spells when you can't seem to

stop coughing? Have you noticed any blood? How much? What color?

Tip: Ask, "Do you have smoker's hack?" Some patients don't consider that a cough.

If he complains of wheezing, ask:

- When do you wheeze? Does wheezing occur abruptly, at night, daily, in certain seasons, after exercise?

- Do you feel short of breath first? Feverish?

- Is wheezing followed by coughing? Does the cough produce mucus?

- Does your nose itch at the same time?

If he complains of chest pain, ask:

- Describe what it feels like.

- Does it hurt to touch your chest or take a deep breath?

- What brings on the pain? What makes it worse or better?

- Have you ever injured your chest? Had muscle strain? Swelling? Tender areas?

If he complains of weight change, ask:

- Have you lost a lot of weight recently? (A yes answer may indicate he has advanced emphysema or cancer.)

- Have you gained a lot of weight recently? (A yes answer may indicate pulmonary edema or congestive heart failure.)

If he complains of voice change, ask:

- Have you noticed a change in your voice? (A yes answer may indicate pathology of left hilum or trachea.)

If he complains of ankle swelling, ask:

- Do your ankles swell? (A yes answer may indicate congestive heart failure.)

If he complains of chest infections, ask:

- Have you or any of your family had a history of chest infections? Have those in-

fections recurred? Have the infections been treated by a doctor? How?

If he complains of fatigue, ask:

- Have you been unusually tired lately? (A yes answer may indicate possible emphysema or congestive heart failure.)

Before you conclude your interview, be sure to ask the following important questions; your patient's answers may be extremely valuable in assessing his condition:

Smoking history
- Do you smoke now, or have you ever smoked? If you've stopped, how long ago?

If the patient is or has been a cigarette smoker, ask:

- What brand do you smoke? Filtered or nonfiltered? Do you inhale?

- How many packs a day? For how many years?

Document his answer in *pack-years*. To do this, multiply number of packs smoked per day by the number of years he's smoked; for example, two packs per day times 20 years equals 40 pack-years.

Occupational history
- Does your present job involve exposure to dust, fumes, asbestos, or chemicals? Have you ever had such a job?

Tip: If the patient's a farmer, ask him *what kind* of farming he does; some agricultural products may cause respiratory irritation.

Recent travel
- Have you traveled recently? Where? (His answer may suggest he's been exposed to a foreign pathogen or toxin.)

Family history
- Do you or any of your family members have a history of allergies? Asthma? Bronchitis? Emphysema? Cancer? Tuberculosis?

Chest assessment

Inspection

To properly assess your patient's respiratory function, you must examine his lungs, using the following skills: inspection, palpation, percussion, and auscultation.

Study the following pages for tips on how to do a chest assessment. And remember to prepare your patient for the examination by observing these guidelines:

• Help him relax. Take time to explain exactly what you're going to do and how long it will take. Answer any questions he has. Don't rush.

• Make sure the examining room is well lighted, warm, and quiet.

• Ask your patient to remain in a sitting position, and have him strip to the waist. Be sure to provide a drape or gown for female patients.

To properly inspect a patient, look at everything, including his behavior. Examine your patient from head to toe, and document your initial findings on his chart. *Remember:* Inspection is an ongoing process. Documenting your initial findings will allow other health care professionals to make later comparisons.

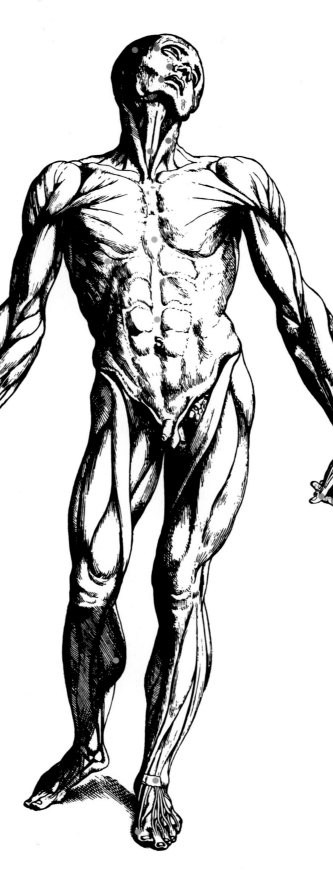

HEAD AND NECK

Mental state
• Delirium, confusion, or hallucinations: May mean hypercarbia or severe hypoxia. *Caution:* With elderly patients, don't attribute disorientation to age.
• Fearfulness: Seen in patients with acute respiratory distress. They're usually restless, with an anxious expression.

Color
• Pallor: May indicate anemia or hypotension.
• Flushing: May mean patient is retaining carbon dioxide.
• Cyanosis of the buccal mu-

CHEST

General observations
• Scars: May mean patient's had surgery.
• Anterior-posterior diameter of chest: Should be smaller than the lateral diameter. *Remember:* Chest tends to become barrel-shaped with lung disease.
• Sternum: Should be located midline anterior, giving rise to a visible projection known as the Angle of Louis.

Chest movement
• Inspiratory intercostal retractions: Occurs in patients with COPD, asthma, or pulmonary fibrosis. *Note:* Sudden, violent intercostal and

EXTREMITIES

Skin
• Elevated temperature: Suggests infection.
• Diaphoresis or clamminess: May mean hypoxia or decreased blood pressure.
• Lack of turgor: Indicates dehydration.

Fingers and toes
• Clubbing: Associated with patients who have COPD, tuberculosis, or chronic hypoxia. *Remember:* Clubbing's divided in three stages —

cosa and lips: May indicate hypoxia, although anemia, if present, may interfere with recognition. Peripheral cyanosis may indicate vascular changes. *Remember:* When patient has dark skin, check the soles of his feet and the palms of his hands for duskiness.
- Pink skin: Seen in patients with pure emphysema. Patient usually thin, with cardiac enlargement and sparse sputum production.
- Ruddy skin with blue overtones: Seen in patients with pure chronic bronchitis.

Patient usually heavyset, with ankle edema and distended neck veins.

Eyes
- Engorged veins, swollen optic discs, or papilledema: May mean patient is retaining carbon dioxide.

Lips
- Pursed lips: Seen in patients with COPD. Breathing out through pursed lips keeps airways open longer during exhalation and helps remove carbon dioxide. Patient can then inspire more oxygen.

- Circumoral cyanosis (a bluish or dusky ring, circling the mouth): May mean the patient has hypoxia.

Nose
- Nasal flaring: May mean respiratory distress, specifically in infants. May or may not be accompanied by expiratory grunt.
- Nasal polyps: May interfere with respirations.
- Red, swollen nose: May mean allergies.

Neck
- Retraction of accessory mus-

cles: May indicate respiratory distress, especially in patients with COPD or asthma.
- Vein engorgement: May suggest high venous pressure. Most common in patients with COPD or cor pulmonale.
- Trachea position: Should be equidistant from heads of clavicles. With tension pneumothorax or large pleural effusion, the trachea will shift *away* from the involved side. With atelectasis, the trachea may shift *toward* the affected side.

neck retractions can be caused by airway obstruction; for example, aspiration of foreign body.
- Inspiratory intercostal bulges: May mean aneurysm, tumor, or cardiac enlargement.
- Use of accessory muscles during respiration: Suggests respiratory distress. Seen in patients with COPD and asthma.
- Localized expiratory bulging: Commonly associated with flail chest.
- Abdominal breathing: Seen in patients with COPD. During exhalation, patient must retract abdominal muscles to force trapped air from alveoli.

This is the patient's unknowing attempt to use his diaphragm to breathe. Teach him the correct way to do diaphragmatic breathing. For full instructions on how to do this, see the patient teaching aid on page 119.

Sternal abnormalities
If severe, any of the following can inhibit respiration and ventilation:
- Pigeon chest: Associated with rickets or emphysema. In this condition, a softening of the ribs causes the sternum to protrude anteriorly.
- Barrel chest: Occurs with emphysema or asthma.

Anterior-posterior dimension of the chest enlarges. The ribs tend to be more horizontal than sloped. No bulges. No depression.
- Funnel chest: Seen in rickets. Softening of the ribs causes depression of lower sternum.

Spinal abnormalities
If any of the following abnormalities are severe, they can inhibit the patient's respirations and decrease ventilation to his lungs. In some cases, the condition may be obvious. In others, the doctor may need to order an X-ray to determine the diagnosis.
- Kyphosis: Patients with this

condition display an abnormally increased convexity of spine.
- Scoliosis: Patients with this condition display a lateral deviation of spine, which results in an S-shaped curve. On concave side of chest, the patient's ribs are close together. On convex side of chest, his ribs are farther apart.
- Kyphoscoliosis: This condition is a combination of kyphosis and scoliosis. The patient's spine is convex, as seen in kyphosis; but it's also S-shaped as seen in scoliosis.

normal, early, and late. In early clubbing, the angle between the nail and the nailbed is flattened to 180°. In late clubbing, the angle where the nail meets the finger is inverted to 120°.
- Asterixis: To check, pull patient's hand back toward his elbow. Flapping of the middle finger will occur in patients with carbon dioxide narcosis or hepatic failure.
- Nailbed cyanosis: This condi-

tion suggests hypoxia, particularly if it accompanies central cyanosis.

Legs
If your patient displays any of the following conditions, be sure you ask if he's had any previous circulatory problems. Record this history in your notes.
- Thrombophlebitis: This condition may lead to pulmonary emboli. Check the patient's calves for redness, swelling, warmth, and Homans' sign.

- Homans' sign: May mean deep vein thrombosis. To check for it, seat the patient in a chair. Instruct him to forcefully dorsiflex his foot. Be sure to document any complaints he has of pain deep in his calf.
- Ankle edema: This condition indicates fluid overload in the patient's body tissues. May be seen in patients with COPD or right-sided heart failure (cor pulmonale). To check for ankle edema,

press your fingers into ankle area, hold, and release. Note the impression your fingers leave on his skin. *Remember:* Always document what you've observed in your nurses' notes so it can be used as baseline data. Then anyone who later records changes in the degree of ankle edema will have the data she needs to make an accurate assessment.

Chest assessment

How to percuss your patient's chest

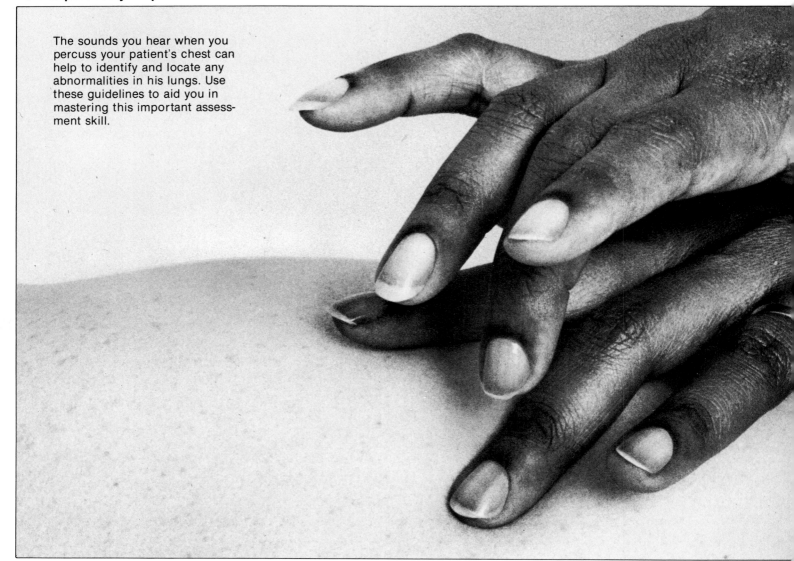

The sounds you hear when you percuss your patient's chest can help to identify and locate any abnormalities in his lungs. Use these guidelines to aid you in mastering this important assessment skill.

PERCUSSION NOTES				
Note	**Pitch**	**Intensity**	**Quality**	**Location**
Resonance	Low	Moderate to loud	Hollow	Normal lung
Hyperreso-nance	Low	Loud	Booming	Emphysematous lung or pneumo-thorax
Tympany	High	Loud	Musical, drumlike	Abdomen dis-tended with air
Dullness	High	Soft	Thudlike	Liver, pleural effusion
Flatness	High	Soft	Extreme dullness	Sternum, atelec-tatic lung

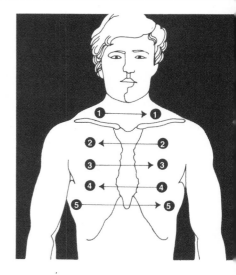

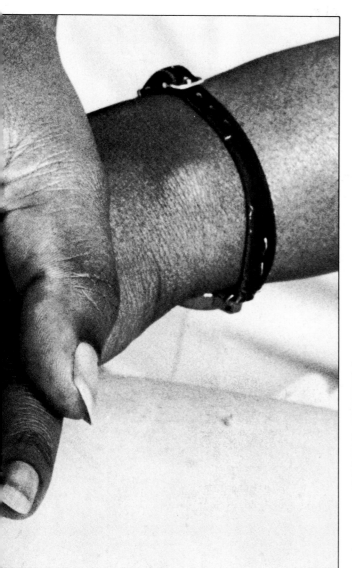

1 The photo on the left shows the proper hand position you need for percussion. Firmly rest first joint of your left middle finger on the patient's chest, but don't let the rest of your hand touch it. Keep the fingers of your right hand flexed and your wrist loose.

With the tip of your right middle finger, directly strike the opposite finger's first joint, just below the nail. Make motion come from your wrist, not your finger, elbow, or shoulder. Withdraw the striking finger immediately to avoid damping the vibrations. Strike once or twice, then move your hands to another part of the chest. Remember, to make accurate comparisons, you must keep your finger strikes uniform.

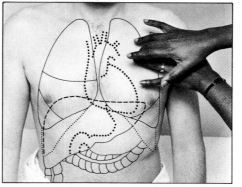

2 Percuss the patient's anterior chest, in the sequence shown on opposite page. This photo indicates where you can expect to find the various percussion sounds. In a healthy patient, the entire upper chest's resonant, except for the area of cardiac dullness. Percuss downward until the sound's dull on the right (over the liver) and tympanic on the left (over the stomach). Document any abnormal findings in your notes.

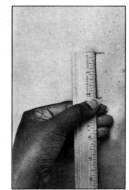

3 Next, percuss the patient's posterior chest, following the sequence as shown below. Percuss symmetrically down the chest wall, making a side-to-side comparison. Do the lungs sound dull? They may be consolidated or filled with fluid. Hyperresonant? They may have large air pockets. Document findings, noting location and quality of any abnormal sound.

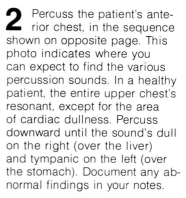

4 Mark the spots on the chest where the sounds change from resonant to dull, both on expiration and on deep inspiration. The distance between them, which is the diaphragmatic excursion, should measure about 3 to 5 cm and should be equal bilaterally.

5 Finally, ask your patient to rest his forearm on his head while you percuss his lateral chest. Start at the axilla, and continue down the chest wall at 2'' intervals. Percuss both sides, keeping the finger strikes uniform. Document your findings in your nurses' notes. *Remember:* For best results, always percuss *between* your patient's ribs, not directly over them.

Follow the sequence shown at left to percuss your patient's anterior chest.

Follow the sequence shown at right to percuss your patient's posterior chest.

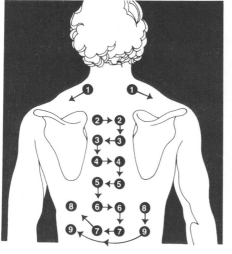

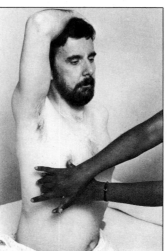

Chest assessment

How to palpate your patient's chest

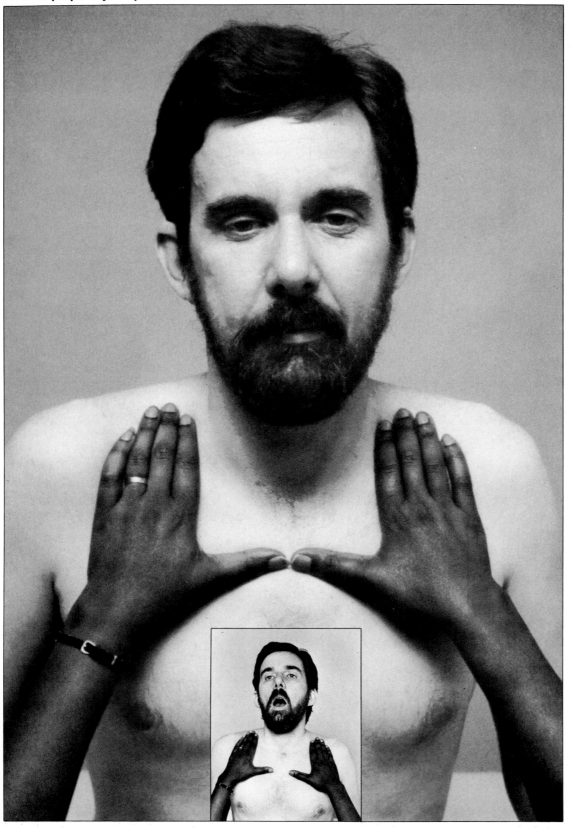

1 *To palpate your patient's chest correctly, check your patient's chest for symmetric expansion and tactile fremitus (the vibration you can feel when the patient speaks). Here's how:* Palpate his upper anterior chest wall. To do this, face the patient, and place your hands on either side of his neck. Rest your palms on his upper chest, and spread your fingers over his shoulders. Extend your thumbs until they meet at midline.

[Inset] Now, ask the patient to inhale deeply. As he does, let your palms move freely, but keep your fingers firmly arched over his shoulders. Watch how your thumbs move. Be alert for asymmetric motion, which may indicate a lesion in one of the lung's upper lobes.

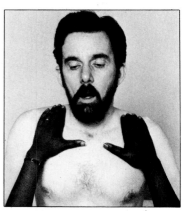

2 A unilateral lag may indicate the patient has a lesion or thickening of the pleura, atelectasis, a pneumothorax, an obstruction of a major bronchus, a misplaced endotracheal tube, or pain on the affected side.

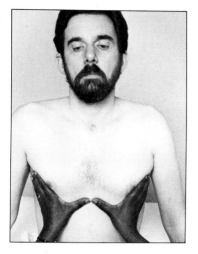

3 To examine your patient's anterior midchest excursion, place your hands on the sides of his chest, dragging the skin until your thumbs meet at midline over his sternum. Your thumbs should come to rest at midline, sixth-rib level.

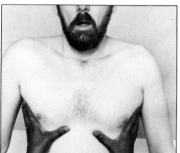

4 Tell the patient to inhale deeply; let your hands follow the chest's excursion. Again, watch for unilateral lag, which may indicate a lesion of affected lobe. Be sure to document your observations.

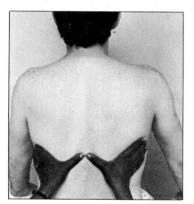

5 Now, examine the patient's posterior lower chest. To do this, stand behind him, and place your hands as shown in the photo. Constrict the chest enough to create a skin fold.

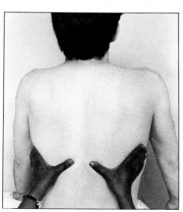

6 Ask the patient to inhale deeply; follow the movement of his chest with your hands. Your parting thumbs serve as a marker. If all's well, they'll be equidistant from the starting point when the patient fully expands his chest.

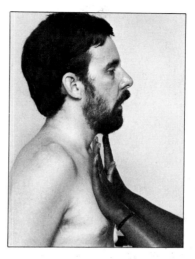

7 Now, palpate your patient's chest for tactile fremitus. One way to do this, place your open palm flat against the patient's chest, as shown, but don't touch his chest with your fingers. Ask the patient to repeat a resonant phrase, like "ninety-nine" or "blue moon," as you systematically move your hand over his chest. If all's well, you'll feel vibrations of equal intensity on either side of his chest.

Normally, you'll feel fremitus in the upper chest, close to the bronchi. You should feel little or no fremitus in the lower chest.

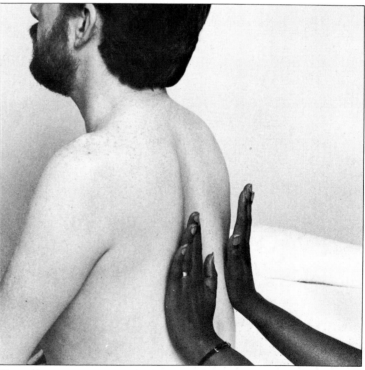

8 Continue to palpate for fremitus, following the sequence shown for percussion, on page 16. Then, repeat the procedure on the patient's posterior chest. Remember these two points when you palpate for fremitus:

If vibrations increase in intensity, the patient may have tissue consolidation on the affected side.

If vibrations decrease in intensity, the patient may have emphysema, pneumothorax, or pleural effusion.

As you palpate, watch for tender areas as well as any abnormal lumps or masses. Document your observations in your nurses' notes.

Also stay alert for subcutaneous emphysema, which may occur around a tracheostomy or a pneumothorax. Suspect it when you feel something like crumpled cellophane under the patient's skin. Subcutaneous emphysema is caused by air leaking into surrounding tissue.

Chest assessment

Auscultation

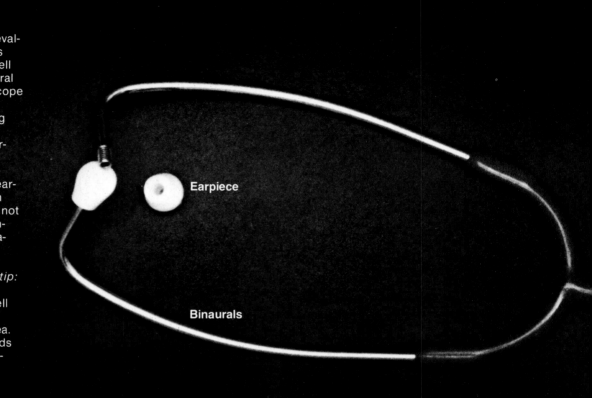

Auscultation of your patient's chest helps you evaluate the condition of his airways and lungs, as well as the surrounding pleural space. Use the stethoscope to amplify his breath sounds. On the following pages, you'll find charts that tell you how to interpret them.

For best results, make sure the stethoscope's earpieces fit snugly enough to prevent air leaks, but not so tightly that they're uncomfortable. Use the diaphragm side of the chestpiece to listen for breath sounds. *Nursing tip:* If your patient's a child, you may find that the bell works better, because it requires less surface area. Remember, breath sounds are usually louder in children under age 6.

Earpiece

Binaurals

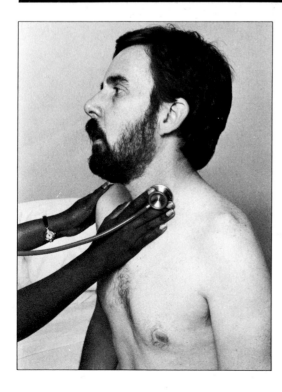

1 Use a quiet room to auscultate your patient. Make sure the room's comfortably warm so the patient doesn't shiver. Place him in high Fowler's position, or have him lie on his side. Apply the diaphragm firmly against the patient's skin and ask him to breathe deeply through his mouth. Remember, if your patient's lying on his side, his uppermost lung will be better ventilated. Keep this in mind when you compare breath sounds. *Nursing tip:* If your patient has a hairy chest, wet the hairs so they don't make rubbing sounds through the stethoscope.

Auscultate for bronchial breath sounds over the trachea and bronchi; they should be loud and high-pitched, longer on expiration than inspiration. *Note:* Bronchial breath sounds heard over the peripheral lung area are abnormal and may indicate atelectasis or consolidation.

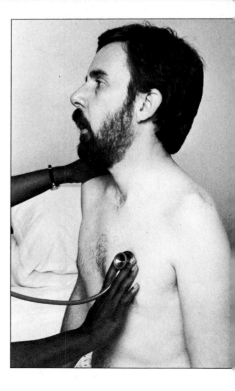

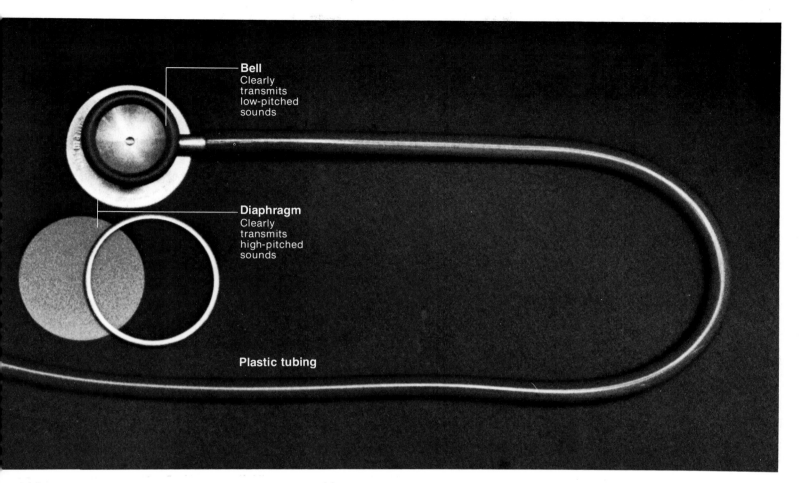

Bell
Clearly
transmits
low-pitched
sounds

Diaphragm
Clearly
transmits
high-pitched
sounds

Plastic tubing

2 Now, systemically auscultate your patient's anterior chest, comparing right and left sides as you move the stethoscope down. Follow the same sequence you used when percussing, and document any abnormal sounds in your nurses' notes (see page 24). As you listen, concentrate on distinguishing between the breath sounds and adventitious sounds such as rales or rhonchi. *Nursing tip:* Suppose your patient has complained of difficult breathing, and you can hear rhonchi in the large airways. Ask him to cough. Remember, some sounds become evident only after the patient's coughed and cleared his airway of secretions.

The illustrations on pages 10 and 11 show how the lungs' lobes are related to the chest's surface features. Whenever you detect an abnormality, be sure to document which lobe or lobes seem to be affected.

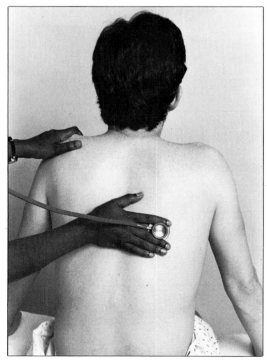

3 Next, auscultate your patient's posterior chest, following the sequence you use when percussing. Note the position of the right main bronchus in the photo; expect to hear bronchovesicular sounds in that area.

Now, check for vocal fremitus (the vibrations you hear when you auscultate his chest). Listen to his spoken and whispered voice sounds. To do this properly, place the stethoscope on his chest, and ask him to say "ninety-nine" or "eee" as you compare the left and right sides of his chest from apex to diaphragm. To assess what these sounds mean, see the Respiratory Sounds chart on page 24.

Respiratory patterns

You can usually determine the rate and rhythm of your patient's respirations by observing him at rest. To get the most accurate reading, don't tell your patient that you're counting his respirations. Instead, pretend you're taking his pulse. Why? Because a patient may breathe more rapidly if he's aware that someone's observing his respirations. Always count for at least a minute. If you don't, your assessment may be off by as much as four respirations per minute.

No matter what the normal rate is for your patient, his respiratory rhythm should be even, except for an occasional deep breath. Study the chart for the differences in respiratory patterns.

Respiratory pattern

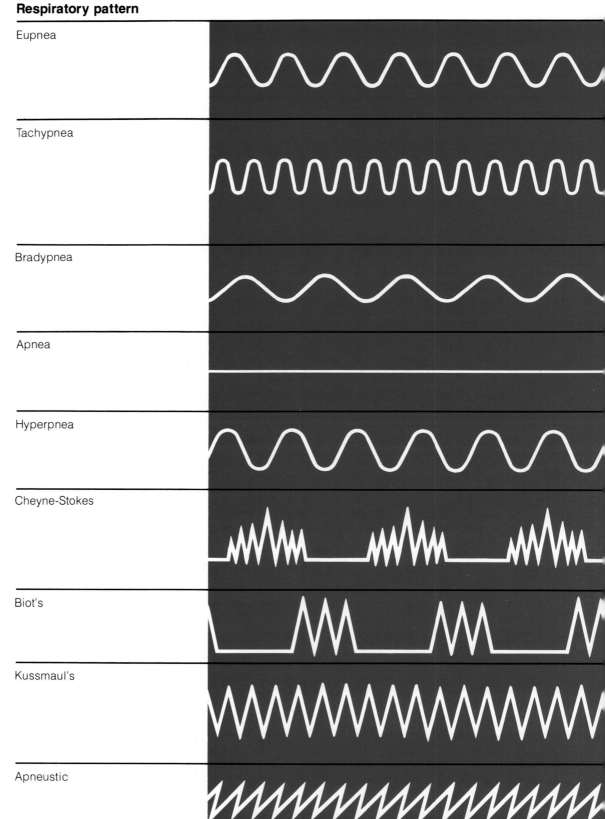

Eupnea

Tachypnea

Bradypnea

Apnea

Hyperpnea

Cheyne-Stokes

Biot's

Kussmaul's

Apneustic

How to recognize it

Normal respiration rate and rhythm. For adults: 15 to 17 breaths per minute; teenagers: 12 to 20 breaths per minute; 2 to 12 years: 20 to 30 breaths per minute; newborns: 30 to 50 breaths per minute. With occasional, deep breaths at a rate of two to three per minute.

Increased respirations, as seen in fever as the body tries to rid itself of excess heat. Respirations increase about four breaths per minute for every degree Fahrenheit above normal. A patient's respiration rate will also increase with pneumonia, compensatory respiratory alkalosis, respiratory insufficiency, lesions in the brain's respiratory control center, and aspirin poisoning.

Slower, but regular respirations. Can occur when the brain's respiratory control center is affected by opiate narcotics, tumor, alcohol, a metabolic disorder, or respiratory decompensation. Normal during sleep.

Absence of breathing; may be periodic.

Deeper respirations; rate normal.

Respirations gradually become faster and deeper than normal, then slower, over a 30- to 170-second period. Periods of apnea for 20 to 60 seconds alternate. Causes: increased intracranial pressure, severe congestive heart failure, renal failure, meningitis, and drug overdose.

Faster and deeper respirations than normal, with abrupt pauses between them. Each breath has same depth. May occur with spinal meningitis or other CNS conditions.

Faster and deeper respirations without pauses. In adults: over 20 breaths per minute. Patient's breathing usually sounds labored, with deep breaths that resemble sighs. Can occur from renal failure or metabolic acidosis, particularly diabetic ketoacidosis.

Prolonged, gasping inspiration, followed by extremely short, inefficient expiration. Can occur from lesions in the brain's respiratory center.

Respiratory sounds

Nurses' guide to respiratory sounds

Breath sounds	Pitch	Intensity	Normal findings	Abnormal findings
Bronchial or tracheal	High	Loud, predominantly on expiration	When listening over the trachea or mainstem bronchus, you'll hear a sound like air blown through a hollow tube.	When you hear bronchial sounds over peripheral lung, it may indicate atelectasis or consolidation.
Bronchovesicular	Moderate	Moderate	When listening over large airways, over either side of sternum, Angle of Louis, and between the scapulae, you'll hear a blowing sound.	When you hear bronchovesicular sound over peripheral lung, it may indicate consolidation.
Vesicular	High on inspiration; low on expiration	Loud on inspiration; soft on expiration	When listening over peripheral lung, you'll hear sounds that have a soft, breezy quality.	*Decreased* sounds in affected peripheral lung may indicate early pneumonia or emphysema. Sounds are decreased because patient's barrel chest causes lungs to be farther from chest wall.

Nurses' guide to adventitious sounds

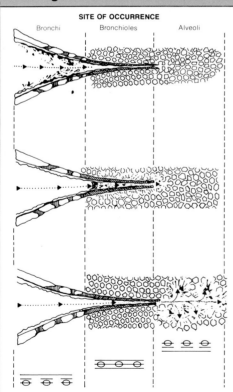

SITE OF OCCURRENCE

Bronchi   Bronchioles   Alveoli

Wheezes, squeaks, crackles, bubbles, and pops
Rales are associated with pulmonary congestion and often indicate imminent heart failure. You can hear rales, usually on inspiration, in the bases of the lungs. The popping sound occurs as air moves through and pops open collapsed airways or parts of the lungs filled with fluid.

As you know, adventitious sounds are abnormal; during auscultation, you may hear them superimposed over your patient's breath sounds. Learn to recognize these sounds and what they tell you about the patient's condition.

Sound	Cause	Description
Rales—fine to medium	Air passing through liquid in small air passages and alveoli	Noncontinuous crackling sounds. (To simulate, rub a few hairs together over your ear.) Heard at end of inspiration, over the peripheral lung. If widespread, usually indicates pneumonia. Also found in congestive heart failure.
Rales—medium to coarse (coarse are sometimes called *rhonchi*)	Air passing through liquid in the bronchioles, bronchi, and trachea	Louder than fine rales. Usually heard on late inspiration or expiration over airways. Heard in bronchitis, bronchiectasis, resolving pneumonia, emphysema, pleural effusion, and congestive heart failure.
Rhonchi-sibilant (wheeze)	Air passing through wet and swollen airways	Continuous high-pitched wheezy or squeaky sounds heard over the airways, more pronounced during exhalation. Usually found in patients with asthma and chronic obstructive pulmonary disease. *Caution:* Absence of wheeze in asthmatic patient may indicate acute bronchospasm with severely restricted air flow.
Rhonchi-sonorous	Same as for sibilant.	Continuous low-pitched moaning or snoring sounds. May clear with coughing. Heard mainly during exhalation. Indicates secretions or obstructive masses in the larger airways.
Friction rub	Rubbing together of inflamed and irritated pleural surfaces	Grating or creaking sounds. Heard during both inspiration and exhalation. Cough has no effect. Found in patients with pleurisy, TB, pulmonary infarction, pneumonia, or lung cancer.

Courtesy: Cherniack RM: *Respiration in Health and Disease.* Philadelphia, W. B. Saunders, 1972, p. 199.

Voice sounds	Pitch	Intensity	Normal findings	Abnormal findings
Bronchophony	Low	Should increase as patient talks louder	When listening over peripheral lung, you'll hear the patient's voice, but words will be indistinct.	When you hear patient's voice clearly and distinctly over peripheral lung, it may indicate consolidation or fluid.
Egophony	High when abnormal; otherwise low	Increased over affected area	When listening over peripheral lung, as patient says "eee," you'll hear his voice clearly transmitted as "eee."	When patient says "eee," it sounds like "aye." Indicates lung compressed by fluid, as in pleural effusion.
Whispered pectoriloquy	High	Increased over affected area	When listening over peripheral lung, you'll hear the patient's voice, but the words will be indistinct.	When you hear unusually clear whispered sounds over peripheral lung, it may indicate consolidation.

Signs and symptoms in common lung conditions

Condition	Inspection	Palpation	Percussion	Voice breath sounds	Adventitious sounds
Consolidation	Less motion on affected side	Increased fremitus	Dull to flat	Increased intensity of voice and bronchial breath sounds	Rhonchi on expiration; medium to coarse rales on inspiration
Pneumothorax	Less motion on affected side. Trachea deviates to affected side.	Decreased fremitus	Hyperresonant	Diminished intensity of voice and breath sounds	None
Asthma and emphysema	Exhalation is prolonged. Patient may use accessory muscles to breathe and have barrel chest.	Decreased or normal fremitus	Resonant or hyperresonant; diaphragm movement decreased in emphysema	Voice normal; varied breath sounds possible	Wheezing and rhonchi
Bronchitis	Variable, depending on amount of secretions and airway edema	Variable	Variable	Variable	Localized rales, rhonchi, and wheezing
Pleural effusion	Intercostal spaces on affected side less defined. Trachea shifts away from affected side.	Decreased fremitus	Flat	Initially, voice and breath sounds diminished in intensity; later, bronchophony, egophony, and whispered pectoriloquy may appear.	Usually none
Atelectasis	On affected side, less motion and lowered volume of thorax. Trachea deviates toward affected side.	Varied fremitus	Dull	Varied voice sounds; breath sounds diminished in intensity; possible bronchial breath sounds	Fine rales
Congestive failure without effusion	Mostly normal	Normal	Normal	Normal	Fine to medium rales, louder on right than left

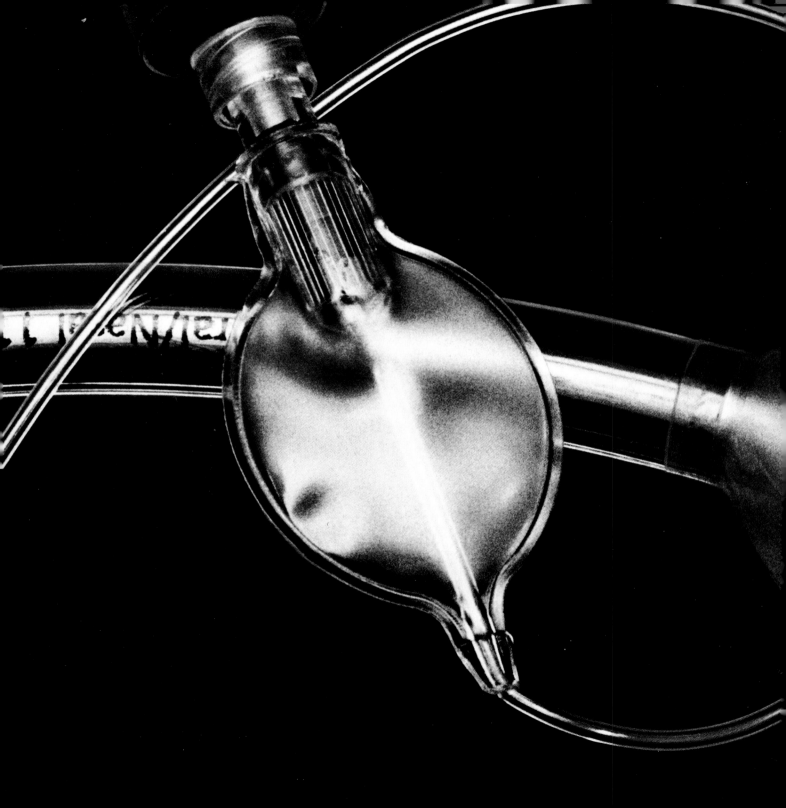

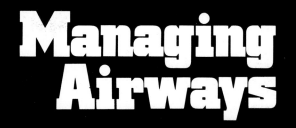

Managing Airways

Pharyngeal airways

An oral or nasal pharyngeal airway will maintain an air passage to the patient's posterior pharynx. Is he unconscious? You may find he'll need an oral pharyngeal airway to keep his tongue from falling back and obstructing his pharynx. Does your patient require frequent nasotracheal suctioning? He may need a nasal pharyngeal airway to help protect his nasal mucosa from injury.

What if your patient's had mouth surgery or trauma, making an oral airway impractical? Again, he'll need a nasal pharyngeal airway.

On these pages, you'll find step-by-step instructions for inserting, cleaning, and removing pharyngeal airways, as well as other useful tips on patient care.

Important: Always make sure you clear any possible obstruction from your patient's natural airway before you insert an artificial one. You'll find instructions on how to do this on page 67.

Inserting the oral pharyngeal airway

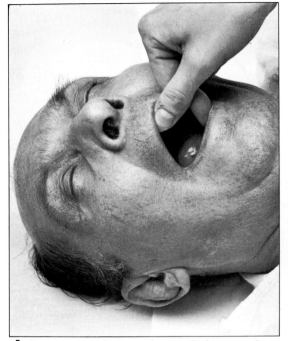

1 *Does your patient need an oral pharyngeal airway? Here's how to insert it.* If the patient's mouth is closed, immediately open it by using a crossed finger technique, as shown here.

Or use a modified jaw thrust. Be gentle to avoid injuring the patient's teeth and gums.

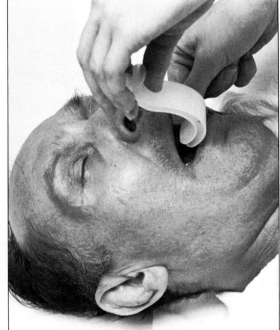

2 Now that you've opened the patient's mouth, insert the artificial airway in one of these two ways. The quickest way is this: Point the tip of the artificial airway toward the roof of the mouth. Gently advance the airway by rotating it 180°; slide it into place.

Don't be surprised if your patient gags at first. If he does, hold the airway in place for a few seconds, until he relaxes.

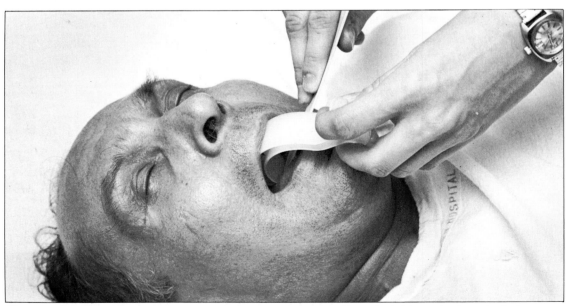

3 Now, here's another way to insert an oral pharyngeal airway. Hold the tongue down with a tongue depressor, and guide the artificial airway over the back of the tongue until it's in position. You'll find this method particularly easy to use with infants, because their tongues are flat.

If your patient gags, hold the airway in place until he relaxes.

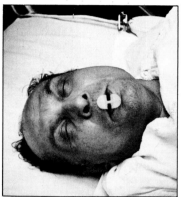

4 Is the artificial airway in place? Position the patient on his side to decrease the possibility of aspiration if he vomits.

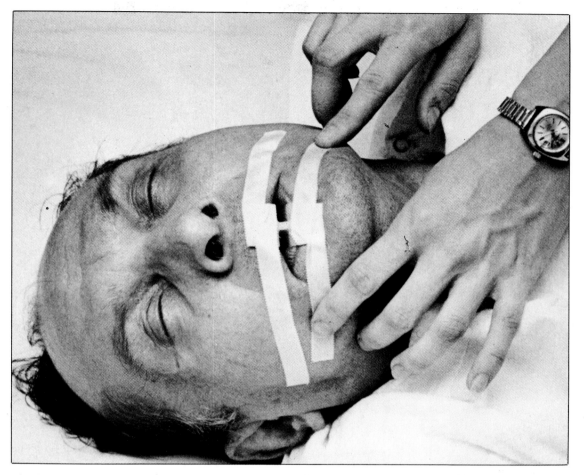

5 To keep the artificial airway from slipping out of place, tape two ½" adhesive strips across the top and bottom of the artificial airway, and secure it to the patient's cheeks.
  Always make sure you've allowed enough room for suctioning the patient properly.

6 When is it safe to remove the artificial airway? When the patient can swallow on his own...or when he's fully conscious and tries to dislodge it.
  To remove the artificial airway, gently pull it out and down, following the mouth's natural curvature.
  Important: Take time to check your patient's gag and cough reflexes. If neither is present, you've probably removed the airway prematurely. *Reinsert immediately.*

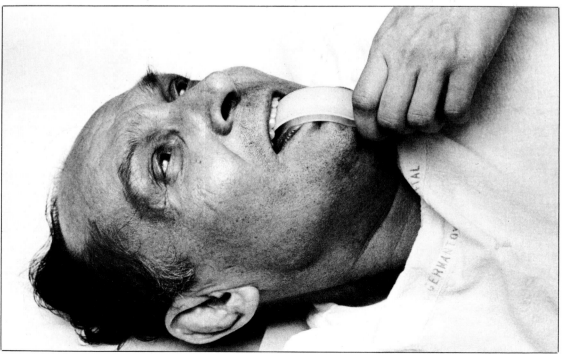

Pharyngeal airways

Using a nasal pharyngeal airway

Suppose your patient needs a nasal pharyngeal airway. Could you insert it correctly? How can you tell if the tube's in the right position? Do you know how to remove it with the least discomfort for your patient? If you're not sure, read the following:

Inserting the tube
Determine the correct tube length for your patient. To do this, measure from the tip of his nose to his earlobe. Mark the distance on the tube. For a snug fit, use a tube with an outside diameter slightly larger than patient's nostril.

Next, lubricate the tube with water or a soluble jelly. Reassure your patient and explain what you're going to do. Then, push up the tip of his nose, and insert the tube into his nostril up to the mark you've made.

Checking the tube's position
Ask the patient to exhale with mouth closed. You'll know the tube's in place if you feel air coming through it. Check the tube's position visually, too. Hold the patient's mouth open with a tongue blade, and look for the tube's tip just behind the uvula.

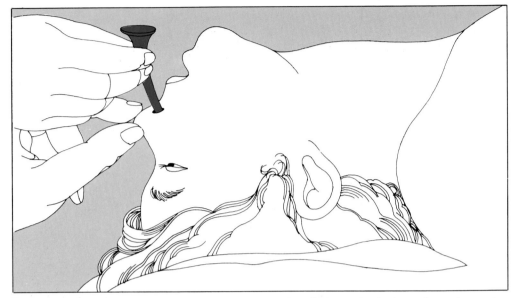

Removing the tube
First, tell the patient what you're going to do. Then suction the tube to remove collected secretions. When you've completed that, withdraw the tube in one smooth motion. If it's stuck, *don't* use force. Instead, apply lubricant around tube and nostril, and gently rotate the tube until it's free. Document what you've done in your nurses' notes.

How to remove dentures

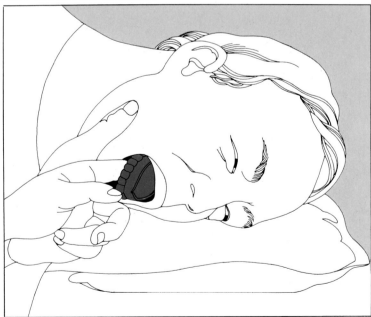

1 *If your patient wears dentures, remove them before you insert an oral airway. Here's how:*
To remove an upper plate, hold down the patient's lower jaw with one hand. Place the index finger of your other hand along the top edge of the denture, just inside the cheek. Gently dislodge the denture. Have your thumb inside the mouth to catch the denture when it falls.

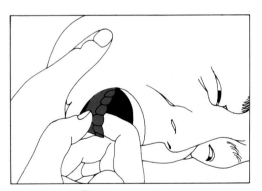

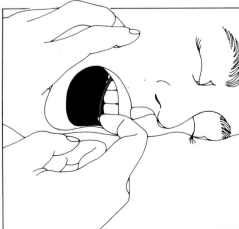

2 To remove a lower plate, hold down patient's jaw with one hand. Place the index finger of your other hand just behind and your thumb just in front of the central incisors. Then gently lift the denture plate up and out.

3 To remove a partial plate, hold jaw down with one hand. With a fingernail on your other hand, gently pull down or up on wire anchoring denture.

After you've removed dentures, store them in a covered denture cup labeled with the patient's name and room number. Document it.

How to give mouth care

1 *Here's how to give regular mouth care to the patient with an artificial oral airway:* First, remove the artificial airway. As you're doing so, place a padded tongue blade between the patient's jaws to hold his mouth open. Rinse the airway first in hydrogen peroxide, then in water.

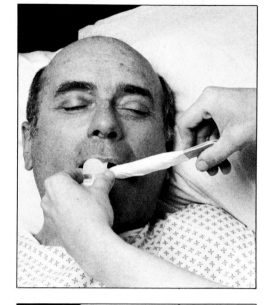

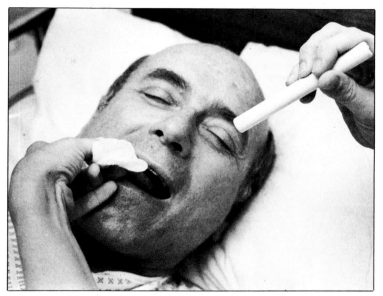

2 Now, use a cotton swab that's been moistened with mouthwash to clean the patient's teeth, gums, tongue, and cheek mucosa.

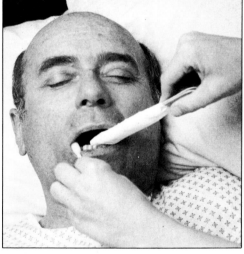

4 Now, use dry gauze to gently hold the patient's tongue while you examine the underside for possible sores. Also, check the color in this area for signs of poor oxygenation. Document your findings.

3 If a cotton swab isn't adequate, wrap gauze around two fingers, and moisten it with hydrogen peroxide. Clean the patient's mouth, as before, with the gauze. But make sure you keep the padded tongue blade in place. *Important:* Never put your fingers in a patient's mouth without a tongue blade or bite block to keep his jaws open.

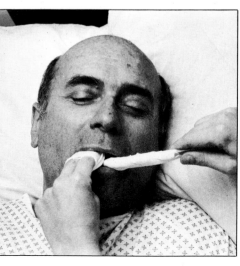

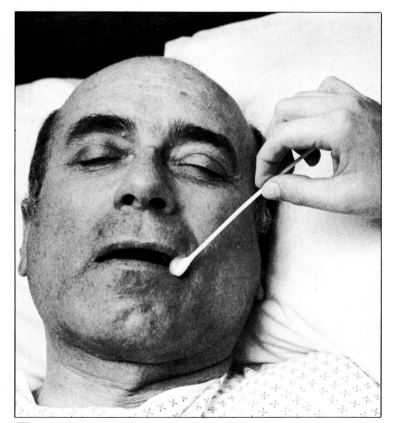

5 Apply petroleum jelly to the patient's lips, paying special attention to the corners. If the doctor orders, you may use antibiotic ointment instead. Don't apply too much, or adhesive tape won't stick. Finally, reinsert the artificial airway and tape it in place.

Airway placement

Nurses' guide to artificial airways

Type of airway	How it's placed	Advantages	Disadvantages
Oral pharyngeal		• Easy to insert • Holds tongue away from pharynx • Inexpensive.	• Easily dislodged • May stimulate gag reflex.
Nasal pharyngeal		• Easy to insert • Allows for suctioning without displacing the patient's nasal turbinates.	• May cause pressure necrosis • Kinks and clogs easily, obstructing airway.
Oral esophageal		• Quick and easy to insert • Prevents aspiration of stomach contents.	• Expensive • Presently available in large size only • Can cause pharyngeal trauma to the patient during insertion • Can accidentally enter the trachea, totally obstructing airway • May cause gastric distention and impaired ventilation if cuff improperly inflated.
Nasal endotracheal		• More comfortable than oral endotracheal tube • Can't be bitten or chewed on by patient • Provides a way to suction • Can be adapted easily if patient requires continuous ventilation • Easily anchored in place.	• Kinks and clogs easily, obstructing airway • Can cause nasal sores, infection, and trauma • Interferes with cough reflex • Prevents patient from talking if cuff is inflated • Tube and cuff can cause tracheal damage.
Oral endotracheal		• Causes less intubation trauma than nasal endotracheal airway • Permits use of a larger diameter tube.	• Kinks and clogs easily, obstructing airway • Interferes with cough reflex • Prevents patient from talking if cuff is inflated • Can be bitten or chewed • Can cause pressure sores on side of mouth • Uncomfortable; can stimulate retching, which may lead to gastric distention • Tube and cuff can cause tracheal damage.
Tracheostomy		• Can be suctioned more easily than an endotracheal tube • Decreases amount of dead air space in respiratory system • Permits patient to swallow • More comfortable for the patient and less likely to become dislodged than the oral or nasal endotracheal tube.	• Requires surgery to insert • Can cause tracheal damage, especially when it's used in children • Prevents patient from talking if cuff is inflated.
Laryngectomy		• Provides a patent airway • Eliminates danger of aspiration • Decreases amount of dead air space in respiratory system.	• Permanent airway • Deprives patient of normal speech.

Endotracheal intubation

Sooner or later, you'll be caring for a patient who needs an endotracheal tube. Will you know what to do? Do you know how to properly assemble the laryngoscope the doctor will require during intubation? Can you fix it if something goes wrong?

In these pages, you'll find the answers to these questions and many more. Among other things, you'll learn new ways to tape an oral endotracheal tube, how to use an Endo-Lok, and how to properly care for the tube's cuff.

_____ MINI-ASSESSMENT _____

Does the patient need an endotracheal tube?

If your patient needs an artificial airway, the doctor will probably choose an endotracheal tube:
• When the patient requires short-term mechanical ventilation or airway management; for example, as he will during many surgical procedures.
• When the patient has a tracheo-esophageal fistula
• When the patient has a serious bleeding disorder; for example, disseminated intravascular coagulation (DIC).

Chances are, the doctor will choose another way to keep the patient's airway open in the following situations:
• When the patient's face and mouth have been badly burned or injured.
• When the patient's an infant (except in an extreme emergency). Why is this so? Because most endotracheal tubes are so large that they're apt to injure an infant's small trachea.

Obviously, the patient who's had a laryngectomy performed can never have an endotracheal tube inserted.

Understanding the laryngoscope

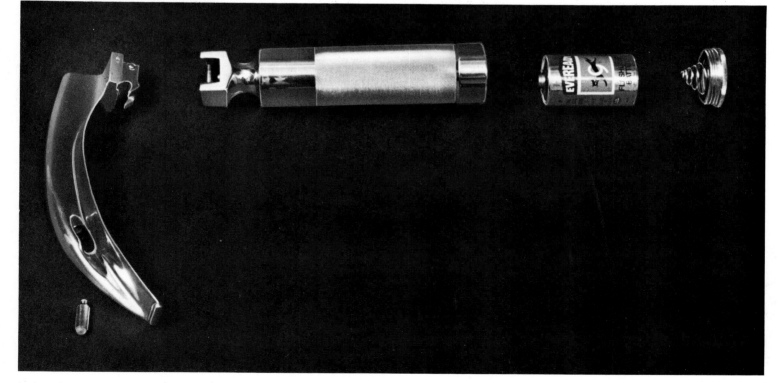

In the photo above, you'll see an unassembled laryngoscope. Putting it together correctly will probably be your responsibility when you assist the doctor during an intubation procedure.

How to do it? We'll show you how on the following page. But first, study this photo. Then remember the following tips that'll help you if the laryngoscope doesn't work.

For example, suppose the bulb doesn't light when you at-tach the blade to the handle. Do you know how to fix it? Follow these instructions:

First, check the bulb. Is it loose? Tighten it. If it's burned out, replace it with a new bulb.

If the bulb seems O.K., check the battery to make sure it was properly inserted. Reinsert it correctly, if necessary, as shown in this photo. If that doesn't work, try replacing the battery. Always keep the laryngoscope in good working order.

Endotracheal intubation

Assembling the laryngoscope

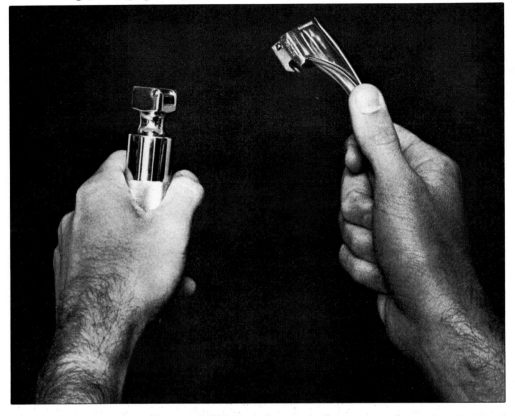

1 *When the patient requires an endotracheal airway, the doctor will need a laryngoscope to ease intubation. Familiarize yourself with the proper equipment so you can have it ready. To assemble the laryngoscope, follow these steps:*
  To attach the blade, hold the laryngoscope handle in one hand, keeping the bar facing the blade. Hold the blade in your other hand with the hook side down.

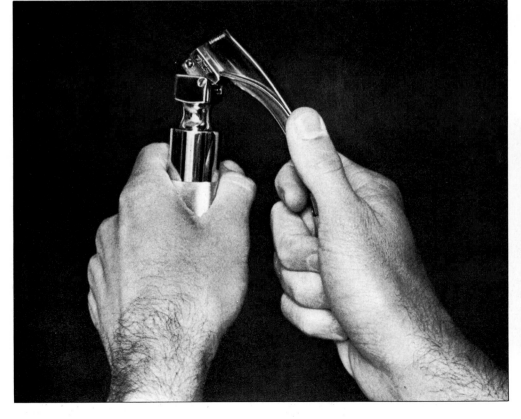

2 Next, slip the hook of the laryngoscope blade over the bar, and pull it down firmly until it clicks in place.

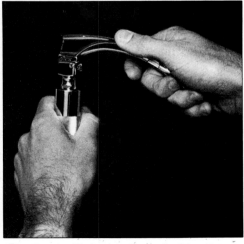

3 Finally, lift the blade up, locking it to the handle. The laryngoscope is now properly assembled and ready to use.

Intubating your patient with an oral endotracheal tube

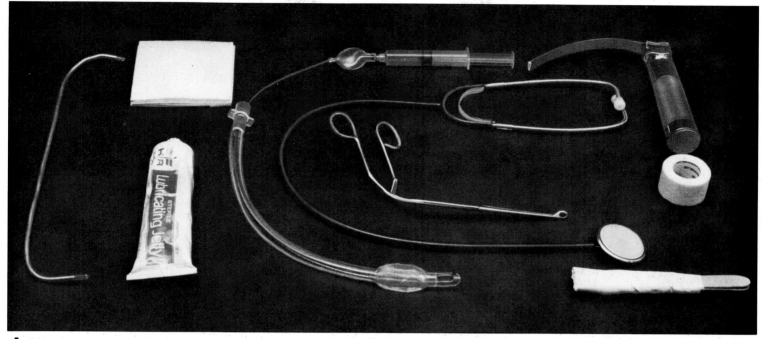

1 *If the doctor's decided your patient needs an oral endotracheal tube, you'll have to assist him. (In some hospitals, nurses are specially trained to perform this procedure; in others, they simply assist.)*

Let's suppose your responsibility is to assist. Begin by gathering the following equipment: laryngoscope with blades, the correct size endotracheal tube, a stylet, lubricating jelly, syringe for cuff inflation, adhesive tape, 4'' x 4'' gauze pads, and Magill forceps.

If you're not sure exactly how to assemble a laryngoscope, read instructions on the preceding page.

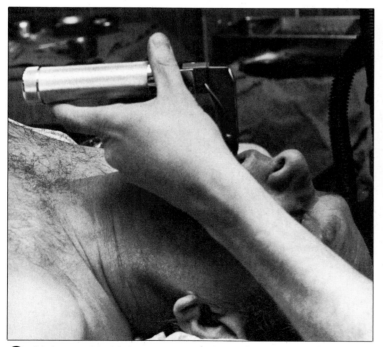

2 Make sure the patient is positioned flat on his back, with a small blanket or pillow under his shoulder blades. This will keep his neck hyperextended, his airway open, and his mouth, larynx, and trachea properly aligned. When that's done, the doctor will insert the laryngoscope blade into the patient's mouth.

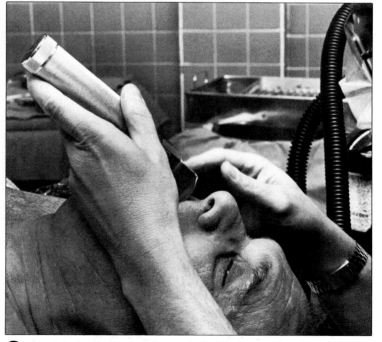

3 Next, he pulls the jaw forward slightly by angling the blade handle upward. This opens the patient's airway even more so he can slip the blade over the tongue into the posterior pharynx, and past the glottis.

Endotracheal intubation

Intubating your patient with an oral endotracheal tube continued

4 Then, as we show in this photo, he'll insert the endotracheal tube alongside the laryngoscope blade, and pass it through the glottis and larynx, down into the trachea. If he has difficulty doing this, he may put a wire stylet into the tube to stiffen and guide it.

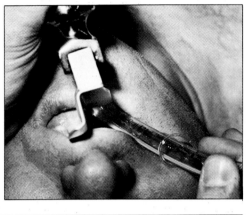

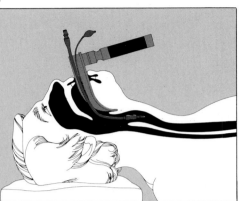

5 In this illustration, you can see the oral endotracheal tube in place. Note how the laryngoscope blade, when properly angled, pulls the patient's jaw forward, holds down his tongue, and opens his airway.

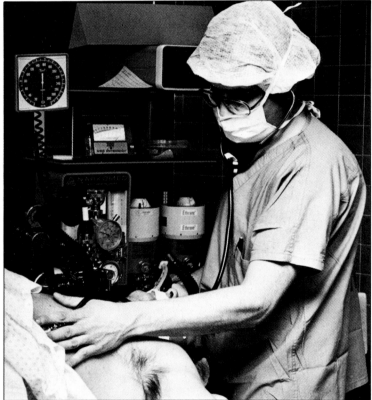

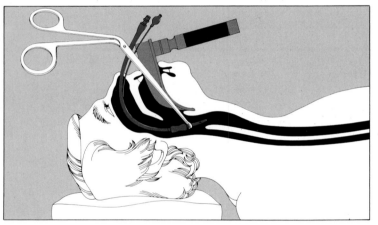

6 Be ready to take the laryngoscope from the doctor when he removes it. After he does, he'll probably advance the tube about 4 cm farther. Assist him, if he wants, by inflating the tube's cuff and auscultating the patient's chest. With your stethoscope, listen for breath sounds on both sides. If they're absent on one side, or if chest expansion's asymmetrical, the tube may have entered the right main stem bronchus. Tell the doctor so he can withdraw it slightly. When the tube's repositioned, auscultate patient's chest again, listening for breath sounds on both sides. If all's well, tape tube, and get a chest X-ray taken to check for proper tube placement.

Nursing tip: Indicate that you want the tube placement checked when you write out the chest X-ray slip. Then the X-ray technician will expose the film in a way that will better enable the doctor to see the tube.

7 Occasionally, a doctor will insert a nasal endotracheal tube rather than an oral one. A nasal tube is usually more comfortable for the patient over a longer period, because it doesn't cause excessive salivation or tempt him to bite on it.

To assist the doctor, gather several nasal endotracheal tubes (in appropriate sizes) and the rest of the equipment listed above. Explain procedure to patient and position him, as shown above. If he's wearing dentures, remove them.

Next, hyperventilate the patient with oxygen, and suction his nasal pharynx. While the doctor applies topical anesthetic to the patient's nose, lubricate the nasal endotracheal tube. Now, assist the doctor as he inserts a laryngoscope blade into the patient's mouth and angles it upward, as we explained earlier, to open the airway. When that's done, he'll insert and advance the nasal endotracheal tube into the nose, during inspiration. As he does this, try to relax the patient by reassuring him. Once the tube reaches the pharynx, the doctor may use Magill forceps to grasp it and guide it into the trachea.

To check the tube for proper placement, listen for breath sounds on both sides of the chest. Look for equal chest expansion as patient inhales. Now, inflate the tube's cuff with 3 to 5 cc of air, and pull it gently to make sure it doesn't dislodge.

Important: Keep in mind that the cuff may have been torn and developed an air leak during insertion. Check for a leak by placing your stethoscope on the patient's neck, to one side of his trachea. Listen for the sound of air rushing through a hollow tube. If you hear this sound, suspect a leak and tell the doctor immediately. He may have to insert a new tube.

Choosing the correct size tube

Is the doctor about to perform a tracheotomy or intubate your patient? Use the chart below to help you assemble the correct size tubing. Then, observe the following important guidelines:
• Always examine the patient *before* you consider tubing size. Look for unusual features or conditions that may affect the size of his nasal or oral passage: for example, overdeveloped neck muscles; a relatively small nose; signs of tracheal or epiglottal edema (wheezing or stridor).
• When you know the range of recommended sizes for your particular patient, select the tube with the largest internal diameter. It'll permit better gas flow.
• The patient who'll undergo a tracheotomy may need an adjustment in trach tube size once postop edema diminishes. Watch for an enlargement in stoma size, which'll indicate the swelling has gone down. Notify the doctor.
• Don't expect to find cuffs on

tracheostomy and endotracheal tubes under size 5 or 5.5; they're unnecessary. A child's trachea is so resilient that it usually seals the air space

around the tube by itself.
• If the doctor specifies a Shiley tracheostomy tube, remember you can only get it in even sizes: 4, 6, 8, or 10.

• Suppose you know the internal diameter of an endotracheal tube and want the French size. To get it, multiply the diameter by 4, as shown in the chart.

Nurses' guide to endotracheal and tracheostomy tube sizes

Age of patient	Endotracheal tube (I.D.)	(FR)	Trach (I.D.)	Size	Suction catheter (FR)
Newborn	3.0 mm.	12	4-5 mm.	00.0	6
6 months	3.5 mm.	14	5.5 mm.	1.0	8
18 months	4.0 mm.	16	6.0 mm.	1.2	8
3 years	4.5 mm.	18	6-7 mm.	2.3	8
5 years	5.0 mm.	20	7.0 mm.	3.0	10
6 years	5.5 mm.	22	7.0 mm.	3.0	10
8 years	6.0 mm.	24	8.0 mm.	4.0	10
12 years	6.5 mm.	26	9.0 mm.	5.0	10
16 years	7.0 mm.	28	9.0 mm.	6.0	10
Adult (female)	8.0-8.5 mm.	32-34	9-11 mm.	6-10	12-14
Adult (male)	8.5-10.0 mm.	34-40	9-11 mm.	6-10	14-18

TROUBLESHOOTING

Coping with problems during intubation

Having trouble inserting an endotracheal airway? Here are some guidelines to help you with unexpected problems:
• *Patient gags repeatedly, making it impossible to pass tube into trachea.* When this occurs, the doctor will probably want to administer a muscle relaxant like curare. For additional information on the dosages, side effects, and nursing tips for drugs like curare, see the chart on page 38.
Important: Remember, any time a patient gets a potent muscle relaxant drug like curare, he'll need mechanical ventilation.
• *Patient vomits while you're inserting tube.* When this occurs, suction quickly. Don't take time to remove the tube and laryngoscope. If you've already passed the tube into the patient's trachea, inflate the cuff. This will keep him from aspirating his vomitus.
• *Endotracheal tube kinks or bends, making it impossible to pass into trachea.* When this occurs, use a stylet to keep it firm. Mold the stylet to match the curve of the tube before you insert it.
Nursing tip: If you don't have a stylet small enough for an infant-sized endotracheal tube, use a straightened paper clip that's been wrapped and sterilized. Always keep one or more of these on the emergency

cart with the endotracheal tubes.
• *You accidentally chip or dislodge one of the patient's teeth.* When this occurs, apply direct pressure to the gum immediately with a sterile gauze pad. Save the tooth or chip and notify the doctor. Take time to document exactly what happened in your nurses' notes.
Nursing tip: To prevent such accidents from occurring, use a plastic laryngoscope blade, when possible. Then, as you insert the laryngoscope, use a lifting motion with the *tip of the blade* to bring the patient's lower jaw up. Never force the lower jaw up with the hook end of the blade. This can severely damage the patient's teeth.
• *You can't hyperextend the patient's neck because he has cervical arthritis or injury.* When this occurs, and the patient's conscious, anesthetize his nasopharynx with xylocaine spray. Then, have him sit upright in bed with his head bent slightly forward. Try intubating him again, but remember, you won't be able to use the laryngoscope this time. However, you'll know when the tube reaches the epiglottis, because it'll trigger a cough reflex. When it reaches the trachea, you'll feel and hear air rushing from the end of the tube. If you don't, you probably have the tube in the esophagus. Remove it carefully and try again.

Endotracheal intubation

Nurses' guide to drugs used during intubation

Drug	Indications and dosages	Side effects	Nursing considerations
pancuronium bromide Pavulon*	*To induce skeletal muscle relaxation for intubation and to facilitate mechanical ventilation.* **Adults and children:** Initially 0.06 to 0.1 mg per Kg I.V. Additional doses at 30- to 60-minute intervals.	Tachycardia, increased blood pressure, burning sensation at injection site, skin rash, sweating, excessive salivation.	• Monitor patient's vital signs and keep his airway free of secretions until you're certain that he's completely recovered from the effects of this drug. • Don't give drug without doctor's direct supervision; never leave patient unattended. • Patient must be ventilated until drug's effect wears off. • Patient must have nasogastric tube because of muscle paralysis. • Instill artificial tears in patient's eyes, and cover them with patches. • Change patient's position frequently. • Store medication in refrigerator. • Don't mix with barbiturate solutions. • Being totally paralyzed by this drug will no doubt terrify your patient; the doctor may give him morphine to relax him.
succinylcholine chloride Anectine*, Anectine Flo-Pack*, Quelicin*, Sucostrin, Sux-Cert	*To induce skeletal muscle relaxation for intubation and to facilitate mechanical ventilation:* **Adults:** 40 to 100 mg I.V. **Infants and children:** 1 to 2 mg/Kg I.V. For I.M. administration: **Adults, infants, and children:** 2.5 mg/Kg. Max. dose: 150 mg.	Bradycardia, tachycardia, blood pressure changes, arrhythmias, cardiac arrest, increased intraocular pressure, apnea, hyperthermia, myoglobinemia, excessive salivation.	• Observe first six precautions listed for pancuronium bromide. • Being totally paralyzed by this drug will terrify patient. To relax him, the doctor will probably order morphine. • Store medication in refrigerator; use only fresh solutions. • Don't mix with barbiturate solutions. • Give test dose of 10 mg I.V. to check for drug sensitivity and recovery time. • Inject drug deep into deltoid muscle when giving I.M.
tubocurarine chloride Tubarine*	*To induce skeletal muscle relaxation for intubation and to facilitate mechanical ventilation:* **Adults:** 40 to 60 units I.V. or 0.1 to 0.3 mg/Kg I.M. or I.V.	Hypotension, circulatory or respiratory depression, increased secretions, decreased G.I. motility, hypersensitivity. Rapid I.V. injection may cause bronchospasm.	• Observe first six precautions listed for pancuronium bromide. • Being totally paralyzed by this drug will terrify patient. To relax him, the doctor will probably order morphine. • Use only fresh solutions; don't use solution that's discolored. • Don't mix with barbiturate solutions. • Inject deep into deltoid muscle when giving I.M.
diazepam D-Tran**, E-Pam**, Paxel**, Valium*	*To relieve anxiety prior to intubation and to facilitate mechanical ventilation:* **Adults:** 2 to 20 mg every 3 to 4 hours I.M. or I.V., depending on patient's response. **Children over age 1 month:** 1 to 2 mg every 3 to 4 hours I.M. or I.V.	Bradycardia, hypotension, tachycardia, edema, cardiovascular collapse, skin rash, laryngospasm. With I.M. injection, possible local irritation and pain at injection site. With rapid I.V. injection, cardiac arrest.	• Monitor vital signs and keep airway free of secretions. • Don't mix or dilute parenteral form with other I.V. fluids. • Inject slowly when giving I.V., allowing at least 1 minute per 5 mg. • Use extreme care when administering drug to elderly or debilitated patients. • Inject deep into large muscle mass when giving I.M.

*Available both in the United States and Canada.
**Available only in Canada.

Endotracheal tube care

How to tape an oral endotracheal tube

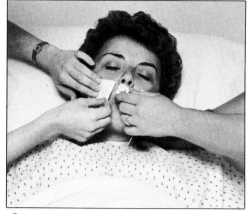

1 *Has your patient just been intubated with an oral endotracheal tube? You'll have to tape it securely to keep it in place. In the following photos, we'll show you three alternate methods of taping. Each will keep the tube from being accidentally removed, or from being pulled off center, which can cause undue pressure on mouth or trachea.*

Here's the first method. Ask another nurse to hold the tube in place. With a 4" x 4" gauze pad (not a spray), apply tincture of benzoin to the patient's cheeks. Allow the areas to dry, keeping in mind that they'll remain tacky. Now cut two 2" x 2" squares of adhesive tape. Press them in place over the tacky areas, as shown.

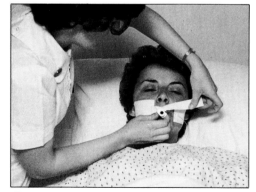

2 Next, cut a 6" long piece of 1" wide adhesive tape. Wrap it once around the end of the tube and cross it, chevron-style, as shown in this photo. Be sure to leave at least 2" tape at each end so you can attach it to the adhesive squares on the patient's cheeks. This method of taping has a special advantage: it allows you to remove and replace the tape, as needed, without irritating the patient's skin.

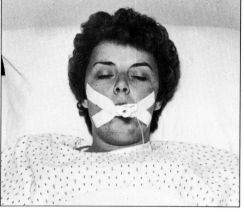

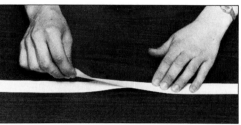

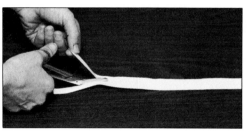

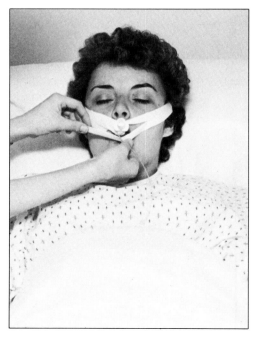

3 Now, here's an alternate way to tape the tube. Cut two 6" long pieces of 1" wide adhesive tape. Take one piece and wrap it criss-cross around the tube, leaving at least 2" tape at each end. Extend the tape ends upward, and press them to the patient's cheeks.

Using the same criss-cross technique, wrap the tube with the second piece of tape. This time extend the tape ends downward. When you're finished, the tape should look like this.

This method of taping holds the tube especially secure, because it exerts equal stabilizing pressure from above and below.

4 Is your patient allergic to adhesive tape? Use this method. First, cut a piece of 1" wide adhesive long enough to fit around your patient's head. Back the sticky side of it with a shorter length of nonallergenic tape, leaving at least 3" uncovered at each end.

5 Slit the ends of the uncovered tape, as the nurse is doing in this photo.

6 Slip the tape around the patient's head, over her ears. Make sure you keep the nonallergenic backing facing her skin. Use the slit ends of the tape to secure the tube in place.

Endotracheal tube care

Securing the endotracheal tube

1 Endo-Lok features: headstrap, protective pad, bite block with opening, strap to hold tube, support bar.

Taping an oral endotracheal tube isn't the only way to secure it. Instead, you can use an Olympic Endo-Lok®, as we've shown in this photo.

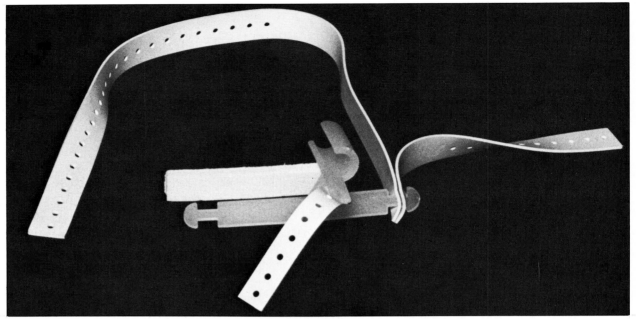

2 To apply the Endo-Lok correctly, follow this procedure. Slip the open side of the bite block over the endotracheal tube so the bite block surrounds the tube. Take care not to jostle the tube as you work or you may irritate the patient's trachea.

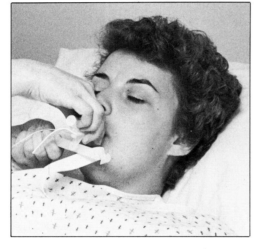

4 Holding the support bar in place, loop the headstrap around the patient's head (below the ears) and fasten it. Or you can place the support bar *above* the patient's upper lip, and loop the headstrap around her head *above* her ears. Take care you don't fasten it so tightly that it pinches or irritates the patient's skin.

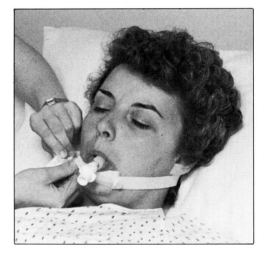

3 Place a foam pad, fabric side down, between the support bar and the patient's chin. Loop the small strap that you'll find at the end of the bite block around the tube. Fasten the strap securely.

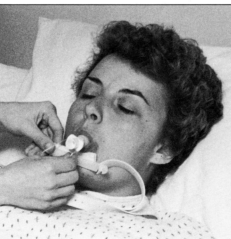

5 Does the patient normally wear dentures? To provide the extra support she'll need with her dentures out, loop the extra strap that comes with the Endo-Lok around her chin.

To check for skin irritation, remove the Endo-Lok every 12 hours. Alternate the way you apply it every 24 hours.

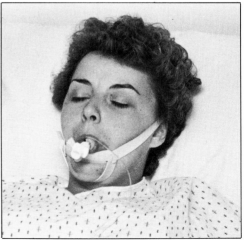

Repositioning an oral endotracheal tube

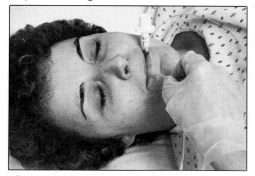

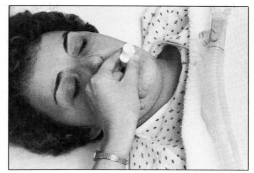

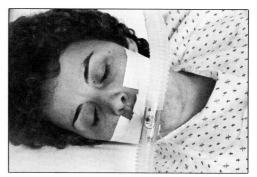

1 *Does your patient have an oral endotracheal tube in place? You'll have to reposition it at least once every 4 hours to prevent mouth irritation.* To do this properly, first disconnect the ventilator or T-tube. Then, untape the artificial oral airway and temporarily remove it. Immerse it in a hydrogen peroxide solution while you clean the patient's mouth. Next, insert a suction catheter, as shown in this photo. When you suction, be sure to wear a glove to keep from contaminating yourself and others.

2 After you've suctioned one side of the patient's mouth, reposition the endotracheal tube, and suction the other side. Don't jostle trachea when you move tube. If you're also planning to suction the patient's trachea at this time, have an extra catheter and gloves nearby. Never use the same catheter to suction both mouth and trachea. When done, clean mouth and lips, and apply lubricating jelly. Remove tape marks with acetone or detachol liquid. (See page 64 for suction techniques.)

3 Then, reinsert a clean oral airway and retape. Reconnect the ventilator or T-tube. Remember, when the patient has an endotracheal tube, you must make sure any oxygen she gets is humidified.
Nursing tip: You may need to suction your patient's mouth once or twice each hour between regular repositioning times. To catch excessive saliva and make her more comfortable, insert a 2" x 2" gauze pad in the corners of her mouth. Keep one end visible so it doesn't fall back into her throat.

How to remove an oral endotracheal tube

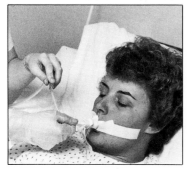

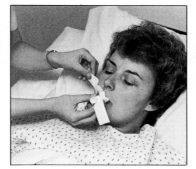

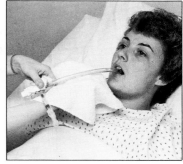

1 *Has the doctor decided your patient can be extubated? If he has, he may want you to perform the procedure.* To do so, first position patient upright. Then suction inside the endotracheal tube. Insert a catheter through the patient's nasopharynx and down into her trachea to suction secretions that may have collected around the top of the cuff.

2 Now you're ready to deflate the cuff. To do so, remove the needle from a syringe and insert the tip of the syringe into the valve at the end of the cuff pillow. Draw the plunger back to remove all air from the cuff. Make sure cuff pillow's flat.

3 With one hand, hold the end of the tube to steady it. With your other hand, remove the tape that's held it in place.
Nursing tip: Have patient take deep breaths as tube is removed, to open vocal cords and prevent trauma.

4 Now you can remove the tube. To do so, hold a washcloth over the patient's chest, and pull the tube out in a smooth, slightly downward motion. Take care not to damage the patient's trachea. Offer the patient an emesis basin if she needs it. Removing the tube may have stimulated her gag reflex.
Immediately after you remove the tube, give the patient humidified oxygen by face mask at prescribed flow. Cough and deep-breathe her. Let her expectorate. Then give her proper mouth care, including a mouthwash. Remove tape marks from the patient's cheeks.

Tube and cuff problems

Problems with artificial airways: How to correct them
Here are some problems you may encounter when your patient has an artificial airway.

Problem	Suspect it when	To treat the patient	To avoid the complication
Tracheoesophageal fistula	• You detect a significant air leak through the stoma or nose and mouth even though cuff is up. • You suction the patient's airway and observe food or liquid in the aspirate. • The patient coughs every time he swallows. • You get positive results from a methylene blue test.	• Feed him slowly in small, diluted amounts. • Suction his trachea through the tube only. • Administer prophylactic antibiotics for aspiration pneumonia on doctor's orders. • The doctor may remove the tube and order hyperalimentation.	• Use a low-pressure cuff and the minimal leak technique. • Exercise meticulous cuff care.
Underinflated cuff	• You detect a significant air leak through the stoma, nose, or mouth. The ventilator shows a decrease in the patient's expired volume.	• Inflate the cuff to the proper size. Make sure you use the minimal leak technique.	• Follow the manufacturer's recommendations on cuff volume as an initial guide, but then use the minimal leak technique. • Measure cuff pressure immediately after inflation, and routinely check pressure.
Ruptured cuff	• You detect a significant air leak through the stoma, nose, or mouth. • No pressure registers on a manometer check. • The ventilator shows a decrease in the patient's expired volume. • The ventilator's low-pressure alarm sounds.	• Notify the doctor, and prepare to change the tube.	• Check the cuff's symmetry by inflating it before insertion. • Avoid accidentally pulling the cuff into the suction catheter when you're suctioning.
Herniated cuff blocking the end of the tube	• You detect a significant air leak through the stoma, nose, or mouth. • You feel an obstruction in the tube when you're suctioning. • High-pressure alarm sounds on patient's ventilator.	• First, deflate, and then reinflate the cuff. Make sure you use the minimal leak technique. • If that fails, use sterile saline to slowly inflate the cuff. Then, remove the saline and reinflate the cuff with air. • The doctor may want to replace the tube. Have a replacement on hand.	• Check the cuff for symmetrical inflation *before* you insert the tube.

TROUBLESHOOTING

Problems with artificial airways: How to correct them continued
Here are some problems you may encounter when your patient has an artificial airway.

Problem	Suspect it when	To treat the patient	To avoid the complication
Carina or wall of trachea obstructs tube lumen	• You have difficulty forcing air into the tube with a hand ventilator. • You feel an obstruction in the tube when you're suctioning. • You note that the patient's blood gas measurement shows a decrease in PO_2. • The ventilator's pressure alarm sounds.	• The doctor may want you to withdraw the endotracheal tube slightly. After you do, trim the upper end and replace adapter. Secure tube with Endo-Lok or tape.	• Make sure you select the proper size tube. • Tape the tubing securely. • Tie the trach ties snugly.
Secretions obstruct tube lumen	• You feel an obstruction in the tube when suctioning. • You notice an increase in mouth secretions (with deflated cuff).	• Move suction catheter to one side to pass obstruction. • Instill saline, hyperinflate the patient's lungs, and suction him with a correct size catheter. • The doctor may want to change the tube, order bronchodilator drugs, or give the patient I.V. therapy. • Humidify the patient's airway. • Perform postural drainage, percussion, and vibration.	• Use humidified oxygen to keep secretions thin. • The doctor may order cooled or heated aerosol treatments periodically. He may also order forced fluids or I.V. therapy.

For endotracheal tubes only

Problem	Suspect it when	To treat the patient	To avoid the complication
Kinked tube	• You feel an obstruction in the tube when suctioning. • The patient's blood gas measurement shows a decrease in PO_2. • The ventilator's pressure alarm sounds.	• Working quickly, deflate the cuff. Then, insert the stylet to straighten out the tubing. • Withdraw the tube, and cut it to the correct length, if needed. Tape securely.	• Slacken the tension on the ventilator and oxygen tubing so it doesn't pull on the endotracheal tube. • Always make sure the endotracheal tube's the proper size before you insert it. • Tape the endotracheal tube securely in place.
Tube in right main bronchus	• You hear few, if any, breath sounds in the left lung. • You observe asymmetrical chest expansion.	• Withdraw the endotracheal tube slightly. Then, carefully reposition it and recheck breath sounds.	• Check the X-ray for proper placement immediately after insertion. • Trim off any excess tubing. • Tape the tube securely to prevent slipping.

Tube and cuff problems

Cuff care guidelines

If you're not sure how to manage the cuff on a patient's endotracheal or trach tube, follow these guidelines:

Keep the cuff inflated when you need a good seal between the patient's upper and lower respiratory tract; for example, when he's receiving IPPB treatments or being ventilated, when he's comatose, when he's in danger of aspiration, while he's eating or getting medication (and for 30 minutes thereafter), or when he's less than 12 hours postop tracheotomy.

Leave the cuff deflated in these cases: when the patient has a one-way valve attachment that allows him to speak; when he has a trach plug: or when he has a T-piece for weaning.

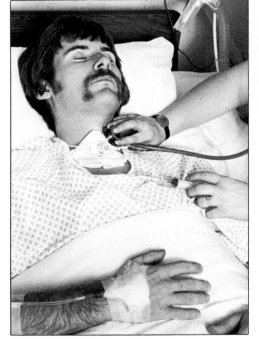

1 To check for air leaks around the cuff and prevent tracheal damage, use the minimal air-leak technique. Here's how: Suction patient's oropharynx and trachea. Deflate cuff by inserting syringe, and aspirating air until you feel resistance. Then draw back the plunger a bit more. If trach tube has a pillow, press it repeatedly.

Now, inflate the cuff during an inspiration. Place your stethoscope on one side of the patient's trachea, as shown, and listen for gurgling or squeaking sounds. If no leak is present, slowly remove 0.2 to 0.3 cc more air, and listen again. (If your patient's on a ventilator, make sure he's still getting his prescribed air volume.) Now, check the cuff pressure. If it's under 15 mm Hg or 25 cm H$_2$O, all's well.

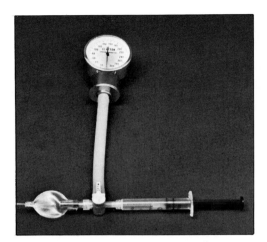

2 You can easily measure cuff pressure with a sphygmomanometer, a syringe, and a three-way stopcock. To do so, insert one end of the stopcock into the cuff's pillow port, as shown in this photo. Insert the other end into the sphygmomanometer tubing, and fit the syringe into the remaining port. Make sure the stopcock lever's in the off position, pointed toward the sphygmomanometer. Inject air to fill cuff. Now, turn stopcock lever toward syringe. Watch for dial to move on sphygmomanometer and read cuff pressure. Make sure it doesn't exceed 15 mm Hg.

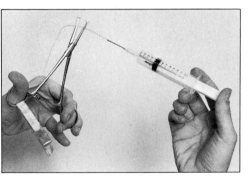

3 Your hospital may have a manometer specifically designed to measure cuff pressure. If you have this instrument, simply attach the cuff's pillow to manometer tubing, as shown in this photo. Then, read the dial to get an accurate cuff pressure measurement.

Remember, on a manometer, cuff pressure is measured in cm H$_2$O. Make sure it never exceeds 25 cm H$_2$O.

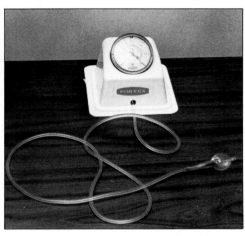

4 Suppose you want to inflate a cuff and you find the pillow has been accidentally cut off. Simply break off a needletip on a syringe with your hemostat, and insert the blunt end into the remaining tubing. Inject air to fill cuff. Then, clamp the tube with covered hemostat, as shown in this photo.

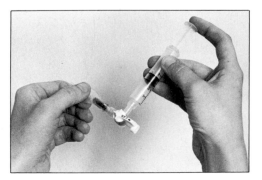

5 What if the tip of your syringe doesn't fit the cuff's pillow port? Temporarily insert a stopcock, so you can inflate the cuff properly. Then, find out which Luer-Tip or Luer-Lok syringe will fit the cuff's pillow port, and make sure you have it by the patient's bedside.

Tracheotomy preparation

If your patient needs a tracheotomy, he'll also need expert nursing attention. Can you give it? On these pages, you'll find clear, comprehensive instructions on caring for the patient with a tracheostomy, as well as an informative guide to the many kinds of tracheostomy equipment in use today.

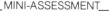

When does the patient need a tracheotomy?
• When other methods fail to relieve an obstructed airway
• When acute edema closes or threatens to close the patient's airway
• When he needs long-term airway management or prolonged mechanical ventilation
• When he can't tolerate an endotracheal tube; for example, in cases of severe mouth or facial injuries
• When physiologic dead air space lessens the patient's FIO_2.

Chances are, the doctor will avoid a tracheotomy in these situations:
• When infection risk is great; for example, when the patient has profound leukopenia
• When the patient needs only short-term airway management or mechanical ventilation
• When the patient has a serious bleeding disorder; for example, disseminated intravascular coagulation (DIC).

How to do a cricoid stab

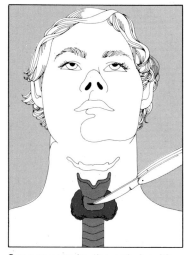

Suppose you're the only health-care professional at an accident scene, and you know the victim needs an emergency tracheotomy. This illustration will show you where to do a cricoid stab. Simply cut or stab the victim's cricothyroid membrane between the thyroid cartilage and the cricoid ring. Then, insert something hollow to keep the airway open.

Important: Obviously, you'd never attempt such a procedure in the hospital. You'd do it only in an extreme emergency situation like the one described above.

How to prepare your patient for a bedside tracheotomy

Although the doctor usually performs a tracheotomy in the operating room, he may want to do one at the patient's bedside. If he does, here's how to help.

First, assemble the following equipment and have it ready: trach tray, sterile gloves, Betadine, sterile water, 3-0 and 4-0 size silk sutures, and a local anesthetic. In addition to this, gather the equipment you need for suctioning during or after the procedure: suction catheters, gloves, and sterile saline.

Make sure the patient or an appropriate person has signed the proper surgical consent form, and get it witnessed. Always check the hospital's policy regarding consent forms *before* you get them signed.

When you've accomplished all this, prepare the patient for the procedure by explaining what to expect. Position him flat on his back. Place a small rolled towel under his shoulder blades to hyperextend his neck and properly align his mouth and trachea.

Remove the bed's headboard, so you can quickly get behind the patient's head to mechanically ventilate him, if necessary.

Make sure the procedure area is well lighted.

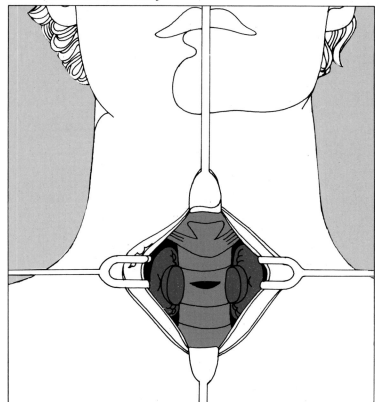

In the illustration above, you'll see where the doctor makes the incision for a tracheotomy. Note how its position differs from that of the cricoid stab shown to the left.

In a tracheotomy, the doctor must first split the patient's thyroid gland and hold it back with retractors. Then he can make the incision in the trachea below the cricoid cartilage.

Tracheostomy care

Caring for your patient's tracheostomy

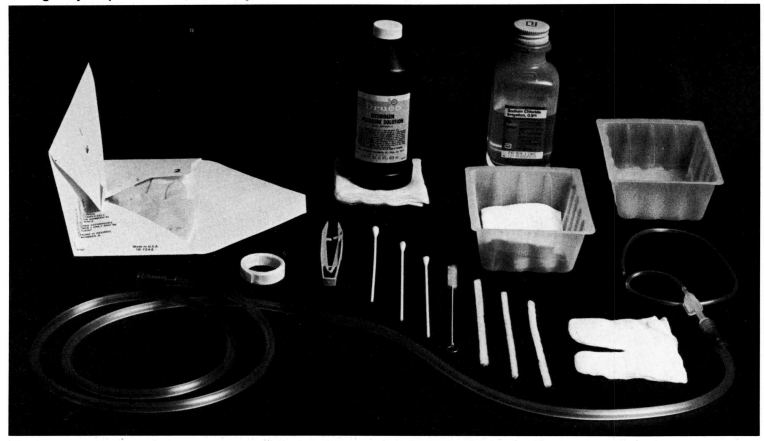

1 *Before you begin, assemble all the equipment you'll need at the patient's bedside. You may want to use the sterile technique described here, if your patient's tracheostomy is new, or if she shows signs of infection.*

Most tracheostomy care kits include the following: two ba-

sins, trach bib, test tube brush, swabs, pipe cleaners, forceps, and trach ties.

Of course, if your hospital doesn't stock preassembled kits, you'll have to gather the equipment yourself. (*Important:* Always keep a duplicate trach set handy for possible emergency trach reinsertion.) Along

with the above items, you'll need: suction catheter, towel, hydrogen peroxide solution (3%), and sterile water or normal (0.9%) saline solution. (You can use the same saline solution you normally keep at the bedside for suctioning. Just make sure it's fresh. Always replace saline solution or water

every 24 hours.)

Now, place the equipment as close to the patient as possible, but allow yourself enough room to work comfortably. Wash your hands thoroughly. If your patient's unfamiliar with the trach cleaning procedure, explain what you're going to do.

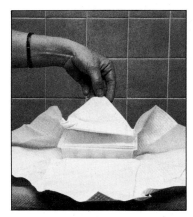

2 Open the kit, as shown in this photo. Avoid contaminating the contents. Don't reach across the opened kit.

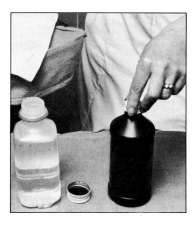

3 Remove the caps from the bottles containing the water and the hydrogen peroxide. To maintain sterility, invert the caps, as shown in this photo.

4 Next, remove the paper-wrapped gloves from the kit. Carefully lift one glove out from its wrapper, touching only the cuff. If you have trouble, hold the paper down to keep its outer surface from contaminating the sterile glove. Then, slip the glove on, as shown in this photo, touching only the *inside* surface.

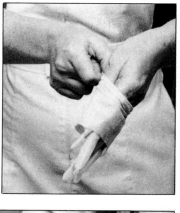

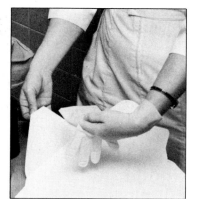

7 Now, pick up the unused glove and hold it, as shown, while you use your ungloved hand to remove the paper wrapper from the work surface. Carefully slip on the glove. Remove the loosened inner cannula by pulling it down and out.

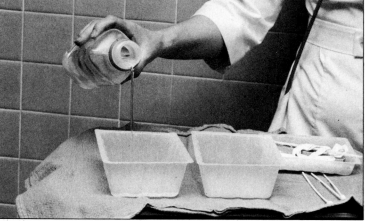

5 With your gloved hand, separate the basins and place them side by side on the work surface. With your ungloved hand, pour hydrogen peroxide solution into the basin nearest the patient. Pour the water or saline solution into the other basin.

Next, suction the patient to clear her airway of secretions. Let her take a few deep breaths before you continue.

When that's done, disconnect any ventilator tubing with your ungloved hand, and rest it on a towel that you've placed on the patient's chest. Suppose your patient can't tolerate being off the ventilator long enough for you to clean her trach cannula. In that case, insert the extra sterile cannula you've placed nearby and reconnect her.

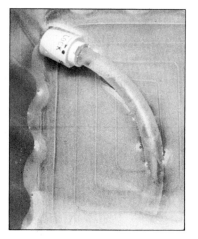

8 Next, immerse the cannula in the hydrogen peroxide solution. You'll see foaming as the solution reacts to the secretions coating the cannula.

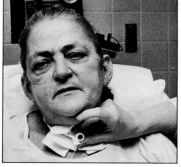

6 To clean the trach tube, you must first loosen the inner cannula with your ungloved hand. If your patient's trach tube is the kind that locks in place, turn the inner cannula counterclockwise to unlock it. Don't pull it out yet. *Note:* If the patient's tracheostomy bib is soiled, remove that with your ungloved hand also. Throw it away. If it's still clean, as it is in these photos, you may leave it in place to protect the patient's skin from irritation.

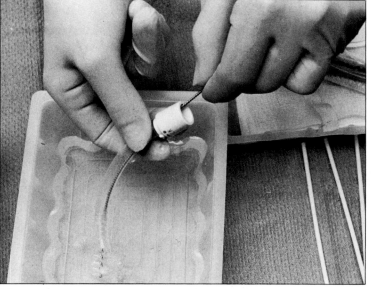

9 Use the test tube brush to swab out the cannula. Don't force the brush. If you can't slide the brush in easily, use a pipe cleaner instead.

Suppose you find you can't clean the cannula thoroughly with the pipe cleaner. Discard the soiled cannula, and replace it with a sterile one from the extra trach care kit.

Tracheostomy care

Caring for your patient's tracheostomy continued

10 Now, drain the hydrogen peroxide off the cleaned cannula, and immerse it in the sterile water or saline. Agitate it for approximately 10 seconds. Remove the cannula from the basin, and shake off the excess water or saline solution. Don't dry it; the moisture that remains will help lubricate it during reinsertion.

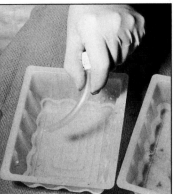

11 Insert the cannula, keeping the curved portion down. With your free hand, hold the outer cannula steady to avoid jostling it. You don't want to irritate the patient's trachea and cause a coughing spasm. Then, lock the cannula in place by turning the hub clockwise.

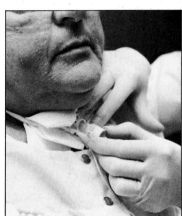

13 Here's how to remove and replace the trach ties. But before you do, remember that in some hospitals you need a doctor's order to do so. Why? Because the patient may cough out the trach tube if the trach plate's not held in place. To prevent this, ask someone to help stabilize the trach plate while you're chang-ing ties, or enlist the patient's help, if she's able. For detailed instructions on how to change the ties, after you remove the patient's bib, read the photo-story on page 51. *Important:* If you do have trouble, and your patient coughs out the trach tube, know how to reinsert it quickly. To learn how, read the instructions on page 54.

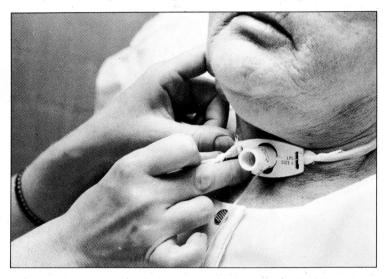

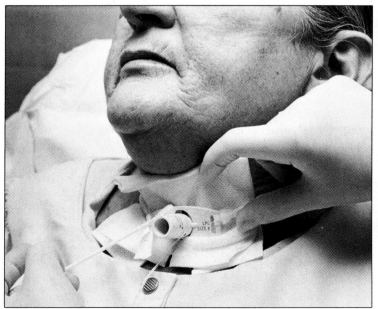

12 Now, clean the trach plate and outer cannula with a cotton-tipped swab dipped in hydrogen peroxide solution. *Caution:* Don't overload the swab with solution or you might drip some down the patient's airway and trigger a coughing spasm.
When you've finished cleaning the trach plate and outer cannula, remove your gloves.

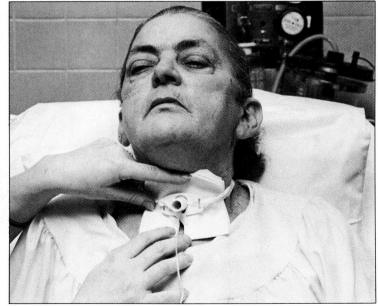

14 Now that you've secured the new ties to the plate, replace the trach bib with a fresh one, as shown in the photo. Attach an adhesive strip just below the plate to secure it. If drainage is heavy, insert the bib from below to provide more absorption under the stoma.

Nurses' guide to tracheostomy tubes

What makes the doctor choose one type of tracheostomy tube over another in a particular situation? This chart will give you some answers.

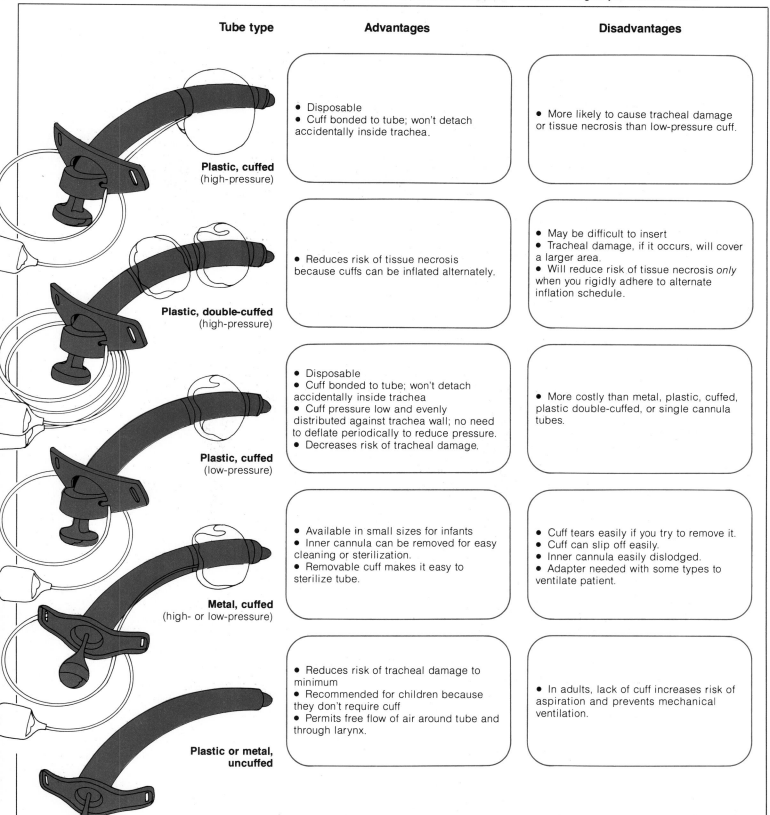

Tube type	Advantages	Disadvantages
Plastic, cuffed (high-pressure)	• Disposable • Cuff bonded to tube; won't detach accidentally inside trachea.	• More likely to cause tracheal damage or tissue necrosis than low-pressure cuff.
Plastic, double-cuffed (high-pressure)	• Reduces risk of tissue necrosis because cuffs can be inflated alternately.	• May be difficult to insert • Tracheal damage, if it occurs, will cover a larger area. • Will reduce risk of tissue necrosis *only* when you rigidly adhere to alternate inflation schedule.
Plastic, cuffed (low-pressure)	• Disposable • Cuff bonded to tube; won't detach accidentally inside trachea • Cuff pressure low and evenly distributed against trachea wall; no need to deflate periodically to reduce pressure. • Decreases risk of tracheal damage.	• More costly than metal, plastic, cuffed, plastic double-cuffed, or single cannula tubes.
Metal, cuffed (high- or low-pressure)	• Available in small sizes for infants • Inner cannula can be removed for easy cleaning or sterilization. • Removable cuff makes it easy to sterilize tube.	• Cuff tears easily if you try to remove it. • Cuff can slip off easily. • Inner cannula easily dislodged. • Adapter needed with some types to ventilate patient.
Plastic or metal, uncuffed	• Reduces risk of tracheal damage to minimum • Recommended for children because they don't require cuff • Permits free flow of air around tube and through larynx.	• In adults, lack of cuff increases risk of aspiration and prevents mechanical ventilation.

Tracheostomy care

Day-to-day trach care

How can you make your trach patient more comfortable? Incorporate these tips in his daily care plan.

• *Help him communicate.* The trach patient who's dependent on a ventilator will be frustrated by his inability to communicate. Be understanding and supportive when he's irritable. Help him find new ways to express himself, by giving him a writing tablet, picture cards, magic slate, or small chalkboard. Allow him time to respond to your questions and remember to speak in normal tones. Try to interpret his body language.

When he's no longer completely dependent on the ventilator, he can speak by blocking his tracheostomy with his finger.

Or you can use a one-way trach valve box or trach plug, as explained on this page.

• *Help him eat.* Should the cuff be inflated or deflated when the patient eats? Leave it inflated unless the patient's had a tracheostomy for a long time and you've assessed, by a methyl blue test, that he can swallow effectively . Give him soft or pureed foods. He may have trouble swallowing liquids. Remind him to take small bites, chew thoroughly, and swallow *between* breaths. He'll find it easier to eat if he sits upright in a chair. *Important:* Keep suction equipment handy in case he aspirates food or liquid.

• *Help him walk.* If he can do without oxygen for short periods, he'll probably enjoy some activity. Keep him from inhaling dust when he walks by covering his tracheostomy with a 4" x 4" gauze pad. Saturate the pad with sterile saline to humidify air.

• *Help him cough up secretions.* To do this, instruct him to inhale deeply and cough. If his tracheostomy's covered when he coughs, the secretions will collect in his nose and mouth. If the tracheostomy isn't covered, they'll exit through his trach tube. Have tissues ready. Also, remind the patient to cover both his nose *and* his tracheostomy when he sneezes.

• If your patient'll have his trach tube in place when he's discharged, teach him how to care for it, as explained on page 56.

Tracheostomy attachments: How they work

	What it is	How it works	Nursing tips
	One-way trach valve box What it does: Enables the tracheostomy patient to speak.	• The valve box fits into the trach tube opening. When the patient inhales, the one-way valve lets air through the trach tube into his lungs. When he exhales, the force of his breath closes the valve. This diverts air through the larynx and enables him to speak.	• Don't use a one-way valve on a patient who has an inflated cuff or tight-fitting tube. Why? Such a patient can't exhale.
	Artificial nose What it does: Provides humidification.	• The artificial nose fits directly onto the tracheostomy tube. As the patient exhales, aluminum foil that's rolled inside the artificial nose traps moisture. Then, as he inhales, the moisture evaporates again.	• The artificial nose is best for ambulatory patients who don't need oxygen therapy.
	Tracheostomy button What it does: Helps wean the patient from tracheostomy.	• A tracheostomy button consists of two main pieces: A short outer tube that fits into the stoma and reaches the trachea; and a solid cannula that completely closes the tube. (The button shown at the left is open.)	• Remove and clean the solid piece at least twice a week. • To give nebulizer treatments or intermittent deep breaths through the tube, insert an adapter cannula through the outer cannula into the patient's trachea.
	Tracheostomy plug (various sizes) What it does: Helps wean the patient from tracheostomy.	• A tracheostomy plug fits into the outer cannula of most small diameter tracheostomy tubes. To wean the patient, you gradually decrease the trach tube diameter, encouraging the patient to breathe through his normal airway. Then you plug his trach tube completely, making it necessary for him to breathe normally.	• To permit a more gradual changeover to the patient's natural airway, deflate the cuff as you begin weaning, or use a tube without a cuff.

How to tie trach twills

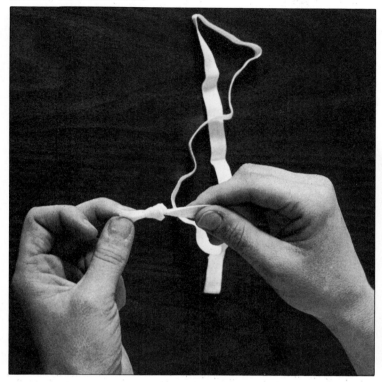

1 *What's the best way to attach twills to your patient's tracheostomy plate? Try this helpful method; it'll help minimize neck irritation by keeping knots away from your patient's skin:*
Remove both twills from their wrapper, and knot one end of each to prevent fraying.

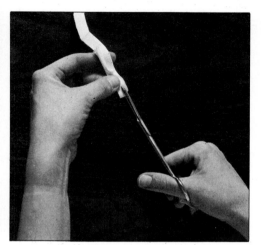

2 Make folds about 1" below the knots you've made. Cut a ½" slit up the middle of each fold, as shown in the photo.

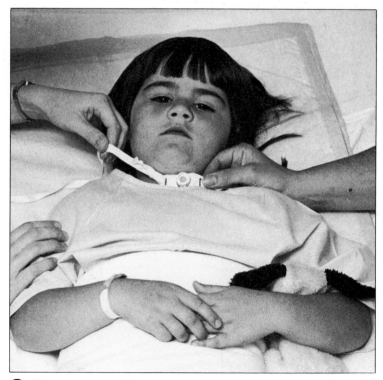

3 Have an assistant hold the tracheostomy plate steady. Take one twill and slip the end that isn't knotted through the trach plate slot from the bottom. Then, feed it through the slit you've made, and gently pull the twill taut.
Repeat the procedure with the other twill

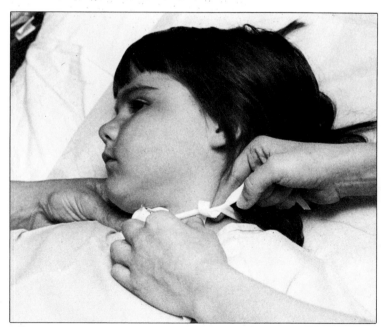

4 Tie both twills together on the side of the patient's neck, *never* behind it. To avoid a bulky knot that could cause irritation, wrap one twill around the other several times before you make the knot. Alternatively, you may use a double bow. Whichever method you use, wrap a piece of tape around the knot to make it more secure, especially if the patient's a child. The tape'll also help prevent mistaking twills for gown ties and accidentally undoing them. Finally, fit a tracheostomy bib in place around the plate. For details on how to do this, see page 48.

Tracheostomy care

How to make a tracheostomy bib

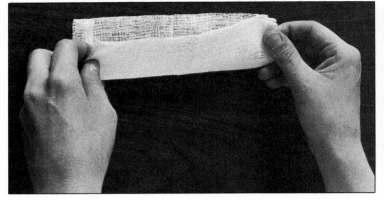

1 *Your hospital may use precut tracheostomy bibs. If it doesn't, or if no bibs are available when you need one, make one from a 4" x 4" gauze pad. Here's how:*
Unwrap the gauze pad and unfold it. Then, fold it in half lengthwise, as shown in the photo.

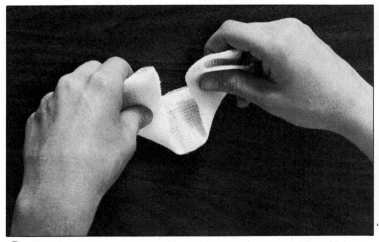

2 Turn back the corners to form a center slot about 1" to 2" long, depending on your patient's size.

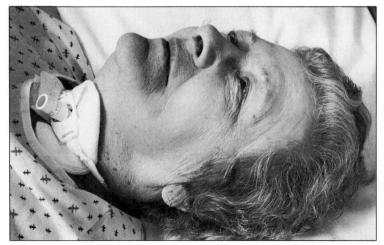

3 Carefully insert the bib under the patient's tracheostomy plate. When it's in place, it should look like this.

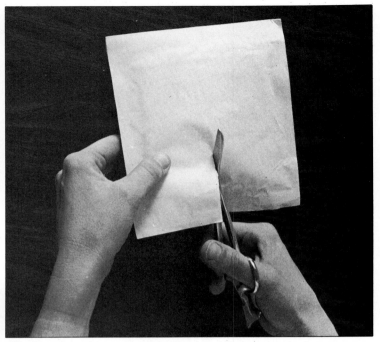

4 If you're using a nonstick, nonshredding gauze pad, you may use this technique: First, cut a slit through the pad and its wrapper as far as the pad's center. Then, cut a hole in the center just big enough to go around the tracheostomy cannula. Remove the wrapper.

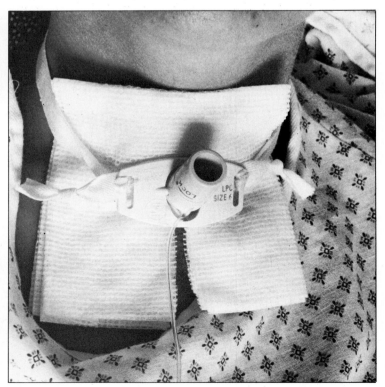

5 Insert the finished bib under the patient's tracheostomy plate. If drainage is heavy, insert from below.

Problems with tracheostomies

Problem	How to recognize it	How to remedy it	How to prevent it
Tube out of place	Trach tube doesn't enter trachea properly during insertion. Instead, it lodges in the surrounding tissues, making it difficult and painful for patient to breathe. This problem occurs most commonly in patients with overdeveloped neck muscles.	• If you can't find a long enough trach tube to substitute for the first one, the doctor can insert an endotracheal tube into the stoma. After it's inserted properly, make sure you leave at least 2'' outside stoma for adapter.	• If the patient has overdeveloped neck muscles, anticipate a problem. Use a trach tube that's both longer and larger. • If the patient's on a ventilator, prevent the ventilator tubing from pulling on his trach tube and dislodging it. Support ventilator tubing with a rolled towel or washcloth.
Subcutaneous emphysema	Air escapes from trachea into surrounding soft tissues. This problem occurs most commonly in patients who are being mechanically ventilated. Inspect for crepitus in the neck tissues. Listen for air escaping around trach tube cuff.	• Check to make sure the cuff's properly inflated. The doctor may want to insert a larger tracheostomy tube. Document extent of crepitus.	• Always use correct size trach tube. (To determine this, see the chart on page 37.)
Pneumothorax	There'll be decreased or no breath sounds on the affected side. In some cases, the patient will also have subcutaneous emphysema, and tachypnea, pain on the affected side.	• In some cases, the doctor will choose to insert a chest tube or flutter valve. Or he may let a small pneumothorax resolve itself. (For more information on this, see Section 5.)	• Watch for subcutaneous emphysema, which may indicate impending pneumothorax. Notify doctor.
Bleeding around insertion site	Postop bleeding excessive. In most cases, a patient will have only slight bleeding after a properly performed tracheotomy, unless he has a bleeding disorder.	• Keep the trach cuff inflated to prevent edema and keep patient from aspirating blood. • Don't administer heated humidity while the patient is bleeding. • Document the rate and amount of bleeding by noting number of saturated gauze pads. • Assist the doctor if he wants to apply Gelfoam to a small bleeder or ligate it. • Ask the doctor if he wants blood coagulation studies from the lab.	• Don't pull on the trach tube or allow patient's ventilator tubing to do so. • If trach dressing's coagulated to the fresh trach site, wet it with hydrogen peroxide. Never pull it off abruptly.
Infection at tracheostomy site	Patient will have purulent, foul-smelling drainage coming from tracheostomy. He may also have a slightly elevated temperature, malaise, increased WBC count, local pain or discomfort.	• Document your findings and notify the doctor immediately. He'll want to order culture and sensitivity tests and possibly prescribe a systemic antibiotic. • Inflate the trach cuff so the patient doesn't aspirate any drainage. • Suction patient frequently, maintaining sterile technique. • Avoid cross-contamination. • Change trach dressing whenever soiled. • Watch for improvement in drainage and document your findings.	• Always use strict sterile technique for trach care. • Thoroughly clean ventilator and oxygen tubing. • Change all tubing and nebulizer or humidifier jar daily. • Collect sputum and wound drainage specimens for culture studies.

Tracheostomy care

How to reinsert a trach tube in an emergency

1 *Anytime you're caring for a patient with a trach tube, you risk that she'll cough up the tube and you'll have to reinsert it.* Prepare for this emergency by having a sterile trach tube at the bedside. However, if you don't have one, use the dislodged tube and proceed as follows.

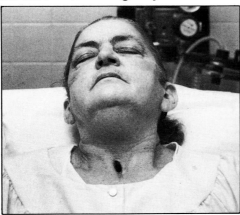

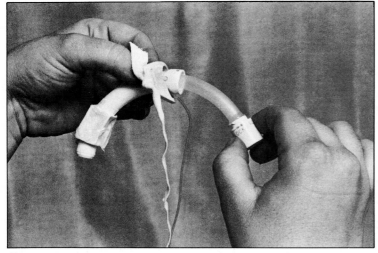

2 Reassure the patient. Then, remove the inner cannula from the dislodged trach tube, as we show in this photo. Be sure you deflate the cuff.

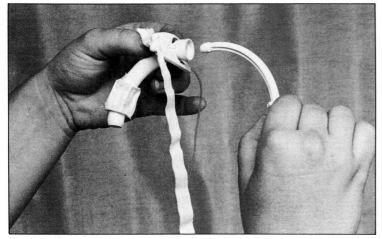

3 Next, take the obturator, which is usually on the bedside table or taped to head of the bed, and insert it into the trach's outer cannula. Then, reinsert the trach tube (with the obturator) into the patient's stoma.

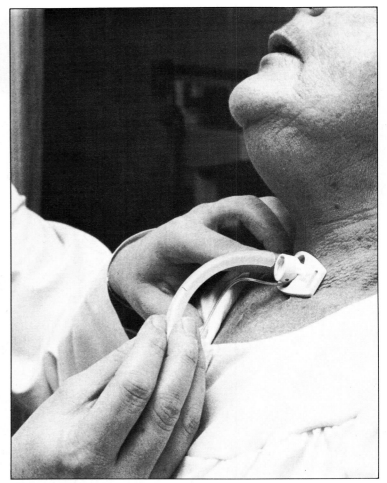

4 Hold the trach plate in place while you remove the obturator. Then, insert the inner cannula into the trach tube, as shown in this photo.

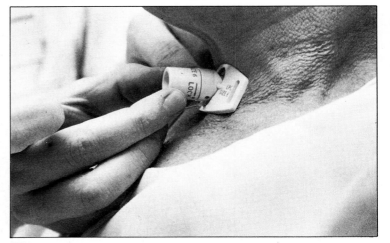

5 Turn the inner cannula clockwise until it locks in place. Chances are, your patient will cough or gag while you're doing this, so be sure to hold onto the trach plate securely to prevent the same emergency from recurring.

6 Now, remove the needle from a syringe, and insert the tip of the syringe into the tube's pillow port. Inflate the cuff.

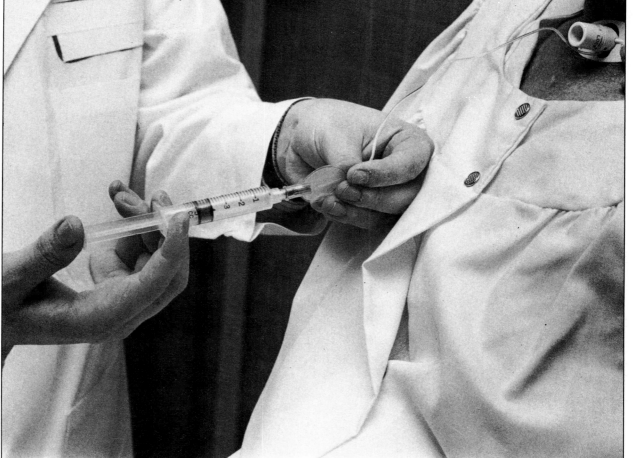

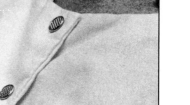

7 Secure the trach ties.

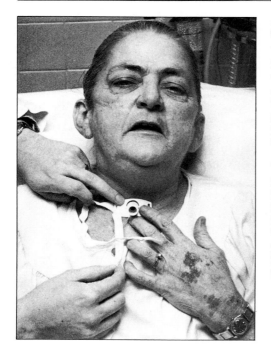

8 Next, put the bib around the trach plate. But your responsibility doesn't end there. Auscultate her lungs to make sure she's getting air. Reassure your patient that she will be able to breathe as before. Tell her that you've firmly secured her trach tube. Take time to stay with her till she's relaxed. When you return to your desk, don't forget to document the entire episode.

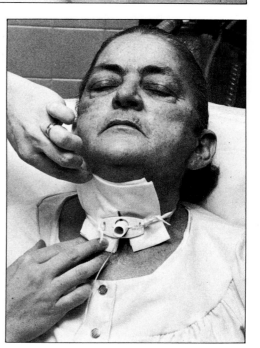

Home tracheostomy care

Teaching trach care

1 *Is your patient going home with a trach tube in place? Before she leaves the hospital, show her how to remove and clean the tube's inner cannula, as well as how to change the entire tube. In this photostory, Barbara Clippinger, RN at Temple University Hospital's head and neck tumor clinic, shares her guidelines for teaching trach care.*

To begin, be sure your teaching area is well lighted, with a mirror available for your patient. Instruct her to wash her hands. Then, using the patient's extra trach tube, show her how to tie the trach twills, cut the bib, and place it properly. (You'll find more information about twills and bibs on pages 51 and 52.) Let her practice these steps until she can do them reasonably well.

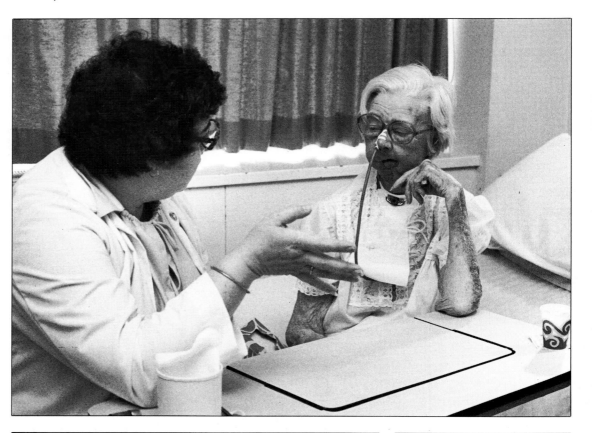

2 Next, show her how the trach tube's constructed. Allow her to handle the tube's parts so she becomes familiar with them. Then, have her practice the turning motion she'll use to insert the outer cannula and obturator.

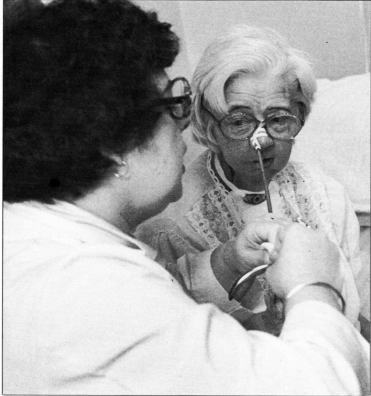

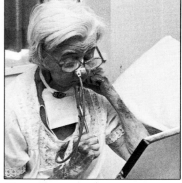

3 Now your patient's ready to remove her trach tube and replace it with a clean one. Hand her the scissors, and tell her to clip the ties to the tube that's in place. Make sure she watches what she's doing in the mirror.

4 Then, instruct her to remove the tube by pulling it steadily outward and downward. Warn her that removing the trach tube may trigger a coughing spasm. If coughing occurs, allow her to cleanse secretions with a tissue before continuing. Put the soiled tube aside.

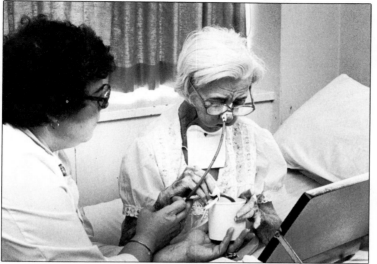

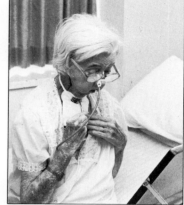

7 Now, tell your patient to insert the inner cannula like the patient's doing in this photo. Be sure she locks it in place.

5 Next, instruct your patient to pick up the clean trach tube, which has an outer cannula, obturator, bib, and ties. To make insertion of the tube easier, have her lubricate the outer cannula's tip with olive or vegetable oil. Don't use mineral oil; it may irritate the patient's lungs.

Tell your patient to take a deep breath and insert the tube into her stoma while holding the obturator in place. Once the trach tube's properly inserted, let her remove the obturator. Caution her to hold the tube in place until the urge to cough subsides.

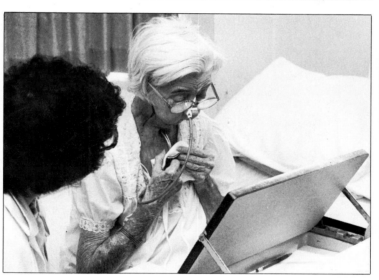

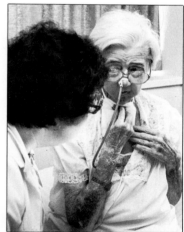

8 Throughout the lesson, watch closely as your patient performs each required step, and offer your encouragement.

Once the new trach tube's secure and your patient's had a chance to relax, teach her how to clean the soiled tube. Here's a good method: soak the tube in mild liquid dish detergent for 10 minutes, and then clean it with a small brush. *Tip:* After your patient's discharged, she can get the special trach tube brushes she needs from medical supply companies and drugstores. However, the small brushes used to clean percolators are just as effective and can be obtained easily and cheaply at hardware stores.

6 The next step is tying the trach tube in place, as shown here. The first few times your patient will need help. Before she goes home, however, she should tie the twills unassisted.

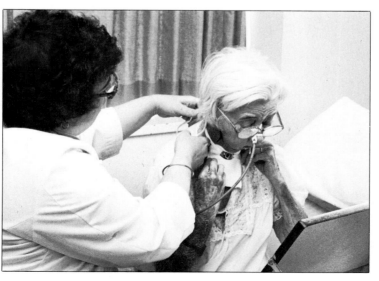

Laryngectomy guidelines

Helping the laryngectomee with problems

Problem	What you can do to help
Inhaled air lacks humidity	Advise patient to: Use a room or bedside humidifier. Place pans of water around the house. Periodically boil water or run a hot shower. Grow houseplants.
Inhaled air's insufficiently warmed in cold weather	Warn patient that he may cough up bloody, dry secretions. Help him soothe and moisten his respiratory mucosa by suggesting that he instill a few drops of Gomenol concentrate 10%* into his stoma.
Smell and taste senses are diminished	Reassure patient that some smell and taste sense will return. Urge patient to install gas and smoke detectors in his home.
Patient fears drowning or suffocation	Warn patient not to swim. Advise patient to wear shower shield (see opposite page). Reassure patient that he won't suffocate if blankets or clothing cover his stoma.
Dried secretions form around stoma	Instruct patient to remove crusted secretions with tweezers.
Skin around stoma gets irritated	Advise patient to apply petroleum jelly around stoma.
Patient's self-conscious about physical appearance	Show patient how to conceal stoma with shirt and tie, scarf, jewelry. With patient's consent, contact local IAL club and ask a member to visit him.
Patient can't hold breath	Advise patient that he'll have trouble lifting heavy objects. Ask patient about his bowel habits. If he has trouble with constipation, he may need a stool softener or lubricant.

*Gomenol was developed at Temple University Hospital's Chevalier-Jackson Clinic, Philadelphia, Pa. It contains 9 parts olive oil, I part Niaouli oil. To purchase Niaouli oil, write D.W. Hutchinson Co., Mt. Vernon, NY 10500.

Preparing the laryngectomy patient for discharge

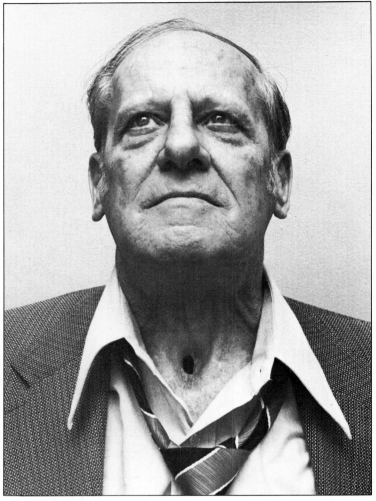

1 *Before leaving the hospital, he'll need not only emotional support to ease his stress, but also practical instruction on how to care for himself. What can you do to help?*

First, do your best to keep him out of crisis. Be sure he understands realistically how the change will affect his life-style. Help him find ways to feel less isolated. Visit him frequently, and encourage family, friends, and other patients to visit too. Make sure he always has writing materials available, and encourage him to use them.

Don't be discouraged if your patient needs a long adjustment time after such radical surgery. But remember that early care and teaching can affect how your patient will cope with later problems. Read the following photostory to learn how to prepare a laryngectomee for his return home. For other ideas, see the chart at left.

As you know, the laryngectomy patient will probably go home with a laryngectomy tube in place. How soon it's removed depends on his body's healing ability and the type of surgery he's had. After removal, he'll have a stoma like the patient above.

Teach him how to care for his stoma by instructing him to wash around it with a moist cloth several times daily, depending on the amount of secretions. Caution him not to clean his stoma with cotton swabs; they have fibers that he could inhale into his lungs. To keep stoma moist, apply petroleum jelly.

2 During the winter, many laryngectomees wear a foam filter like this one to warm air as it's inhaled. In addition, the filter helps screen out air pollutants and prevents foreign material, like hair and food particles, from entering the stoma.

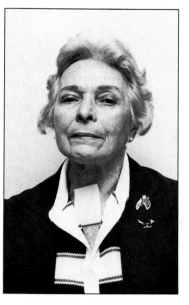

3 To shield her stoma and to cover the filter, your patient may wear a crocheted bib like the one in this photo. Instruct your patient to change both filter and bib when they're soiled, and to carefully clean around her stoma. Help her get the new bibs and filters she needs when she returns home. Tell your patient to contact the nearest chapter of the International Association of Laryngectomees (see information below).

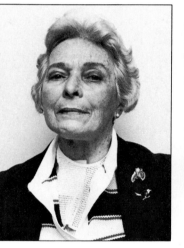

4 To protect his stoma when showering, your patient can wear a stoma shield like the one in this illustration. Alternatively, he can simply direct the stream of water to hit below the level of his stoma.

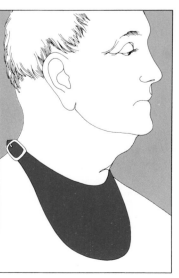

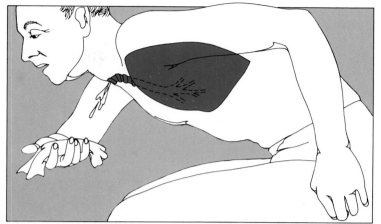

5 This illustration shows how your patient should position himself to cough. If he keeps his stoma below lung level, he can expel secretions more easily.

Nursing tip: To prevent his embarrassment, remind your patient to cover his stoma when he coughs or sneezes.

6 Take time to advise your patient and his family of the help they can get from the International Association of Laryngectomees (IAL). This volunteer organization has local chapters in most states and in many foreign countries. Among other services, IAL clubs provide the following:
• psychologic counseling for new laryngectomees and their families
• fellowship with other laryngectomees who've successfully overcome their handicap
• help in locating qualified speech therapists
• help in locating needed equipment, for example, stoma shields and bibs.

The typical packet shown here is available to new members of the Philadelphia Laryn-gects Club. It contains:
• an emergency I.D. card that identifies the bearer as a laryngectomee
• order blank for Medic Alert bracelet
• a car windshield sticker (in case of accident)
• a portable slate
• background information on the IAL and its activities.

To find the nearest club, tell your patient to write: International Association of Laryngectomees, American Cancer Society, 777 Third Avenue, New York, N.Y. 10017.

You may also suggest that he write for the following free booklet: *Looking Forward: A Guidebook for the Laryngectomee,* Mayo Foundation, Rochester, Minn. 55901.

Suctioning

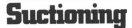

Do you know when and how to suction your patient? This sequence will show you, as well as explain some of the problems you may encounter.

But first, let's discuss how to prepare your patient for the procedure. Keep in mind that he'll probably be frightened, especially if he's never been suctioned before. Ease his distress by explaining what you're going to do and how it'll help him breathe easier. Here are some guidelines to help you:

• Explain how suctioning will remove some of the secretions that have collected in his respiratory tract from illness or surgery.

• Go through a step-by-step explanation of the procedure. Be sure to tell him that you'll be inserting a catheter into his nose, mouth, or endotracheal tube.

• Tell him how the procedure will feel. For example, with nasal or oral suctioning, say something like: "When the catheter reaches the back of your nose, you'll feel some pressure," or, "When the catheter touches your throat, you'll probably feel like gagging or coughing. To prevent this, try to relax and breathe deeply through your mouth."

• Never rush the procedure. Your patient will be more relaxed and your job will be easier if you take your time.

MINI-ASSESSMENT

Does your patient need suctioning?

Prepare to suction your patient any time he's unable to cough up secretions that obstruct his airway. This can happen when:

• he has a neuromuscular disorder that keeps him from coughing; for example, Guillain-Barré syndrome.

• he has unusually heavy or thick secretions; for example, from pulmonary edema or cystic fibrosis.

• he's lost his cough reflex from head injury, anesthesia, or drug overdose.

• his airway is obstructed by an endotracheal tube or his jaws are wired shut after reconstructive surgery.

Watch for these danger signs that indicate your patient may require regular suctioning:

• dyspnea

• tachycardia

• audible rales, diminished breath sounds

• restlessness, agitation

• rhonchi and gurgling over large airways.

Also, listen for the ventilator's pressure alarm to go off. This may indicate that the patient's airway is partially obstructed and he needs suctioning. Use caution suctioning your patient if he's had recent surgery on his nose, throat, esophagus, or trachea. Suction cautiously through his nasopharynx if he has a blood dyscrasia or is on anticoagulants. Never suction if he shows signs of a spinal fluid leak, or active bleeding from his nasopharynx. *Nursing tip:* To detect a spinal fluid leak, watch for a halo around stains caused by nasal secretions.

How well is your patient tolerating the procedure? Watch for these signs of complications:

• bloody aspirant, indicating possible nasal or tracheal damage

• cardiac arrhythmias, particularly bradycardia or atrioventricular (AV) heart block

• cyanosis, indicating hypoxia

• bronchospasm.

Do your best to prevent arrhythmias, hypoxia, or bronchospasms from occurring by giving your patient an increased amount of oxygen before you begin suctioning. *Important:* In cases of bronchospasm, you may find it hard to remove the suction catheter. Don't try. Instead, disconnect the tube connecting the suction catheter to the suction equipment, and let the catheter act as an artificial airway.

After any suctioning, auscultate the patient's lungs to make sure the suctioning was effective. Remember to chart your findings.

What you should know about suctioning

Before you read the next few photostories, review these general guidelines about suctioning:

• Whenever possible, take the time to cough and deep breathe your patient before you begin the procedure.

• Never prolong suctioning beyond 12 seconds. If the patient needs more, first encourage him to breathe deeply for at least 1 minute.

• Is your patient on continuous oxygen therapy? If he is, hyperventilate his lungs for several minutes before and after you suction him. Be sure to turn the oxygen back to the prescribed flow rate afterwards.

When you've finished suctioning:

• Immediately reconnect the patient to ventilator or oxygen delivery system.

• Discard the used suction catheter, gloves, and basin. Make sure there's new equipment at the bedside.

• Wrap the connector tube around the suction gauge to keep it out of the way.

• Document when and why you suctioned, in your notes. (See page 63 for tips.) Describe the amount of sputum as well as its color and consistency.

• Replace saline solutions and sterile water with a fresh supply every 24 hours. Write the date and time you opened it on the label.

• Remember to empty and rinse vacuum bottles at the end of each shift.

How to do nasotracheal suctioning

1 *Doing nasotracheal suctioning isn't difficult, if you follow the correct procedure.* First, gather the necessary equipment: sterile suction catheter, sterile disposable basin, sterile water or saline solution, sterile gloves, water-soluble jelly, a suction device, and a Y-connector (if the catheter you're using doesn't have a control valve).

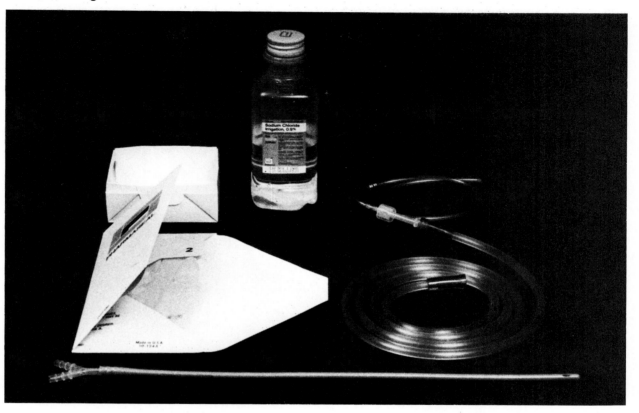

2 Next, prepare the patient. Have him sit at a 45° angle, as we show in this photo. Instruct him to breathe deeply. If he's getting oxygen, increase flow rate for a few moments.

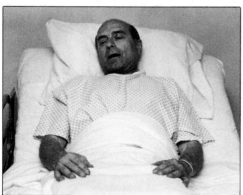

3 Now, pour sterile saline solution into the sterile basin. Pour the solution as shown, to keep it from dripping from the unsterile bottle lip.

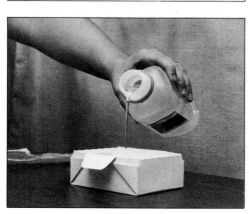

4 Now, slip a sterile glove on the hand you'll be using to suction the patient.

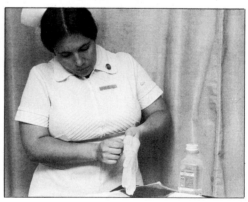

5 With your gloved hand, remove the sterile catheter from its wrapper. Keep it coiled, so it can't touch any unsterile object. *Important:* If the catheter and gloves are packaged separately, open the catheter package *before* you slip on the glove.

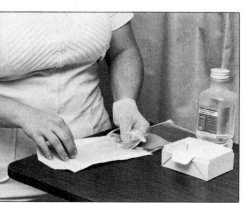

Suctioning

How to do nasotracheal suctioning continued

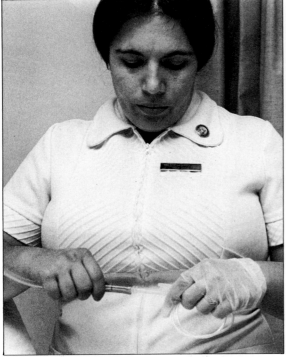

6 Connect the sterile catheter directly to the suction tubing, making sure you keep the catheter in your gloved hand.

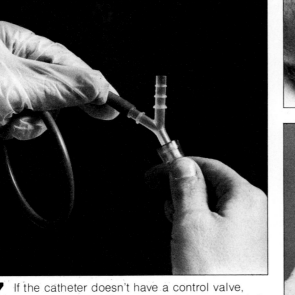

7 If the catheter doesn't have a control valve, connect it to a Y-connector *before* you attach it to the suction tubing. Later, during the procedure, you'll control suctioning by intermittently covering the open end of the Y-connector with one finger. *Nursing tip:* You can also control suctioning by bending and pinching the catheter between your fingers.

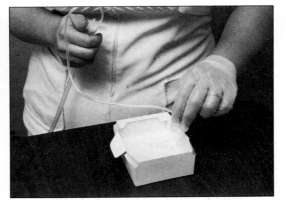

8 Now, measure the catheter from the patient's ear lobe to the tip of his nose. Next, lubricate the tip of the catheter by dipping it into the basin of sterile saline.

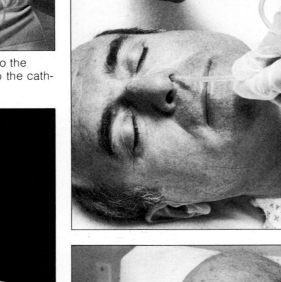

9 Gently insert the catheter into your patient's nostril. Advance it as far as it'll go, but *don't suction yet*. To make insertion easier, ask the patient to take slow, deep breaths through his mouth. Have him stick out his tongue to prevent him from swallowing. When the catheter's in, withdraw it slightly (about I to 2 cm).

Ask the patient to turn his head to one side to facilitate suctioning of the main bronchus on the opposite side. When you suction again, ask him to reverse his head position. Avoid nasotracheal suctioning unless other methods of secretion removal fail. This method can affect the patient's heart rate and rhythm by stimulating the sensory receptors of his vagus nerve.

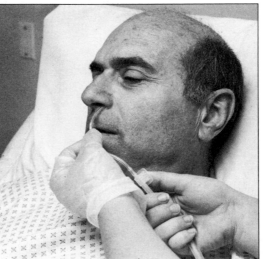

10 Begin suctioning the patient, using a pill-rolling technique to manage the catheter. Use this technique with a straight catheter only. If you use it with an angled catheter, you may injure his trachea. *Caution:* To prevent hypoxia, never suction longer than 12 seconds at a time. Rinse catheter with normal saline solution before you reinsert it.

When you've completed the procedure, instruct patient to breathe deeply. If he's on oxygen, increase flow rate for a few moments. Then turn it back to prescribed rate.

Patient Progress Notes

NAME _Dorothy Bacon_

AGE _80 yrs_

DATE	TIME	NO.	PROBLEM	
5 July 79	2³⁰PM	1C	Pneumonia	S: Patient states she is tired from coughing. She c/o tenderness over the right side of her chest and abdomen.
				O: T-101.6°F P-106 and regular R-25. Fine rales with suppressed breath sounds at the base of the (R) lung. Copious amounts of yellow, mucopurulent sputum obtained when suctioned.
				A: Resolving lung infection
				P: Continue care plan
				I: Suctioned q 2 hrs.(and PRN) prior to repositioning. Mucomyst by nebulizer given prior to chest P.T. at 10 AM and 2 PM. Hydration maintained and antipyretic given x 2. No side effects noted from penicillin therapy. Will send sputum specimen to lab if change noted in color, amount and /or odor of secretions.
				B. McVan R.N.

PROGRESS NOTE FORMAT

S: Subjective data (symptoms)
O: Objective data (measurable signs)
A: Assessment (conclusion)

P: Plan—immediate or future
I: Intervention—nursing action
E: Evaluation—effectiveness or ineffectiveness of intervention
R: Revision—chance care plan appropriately

Suctioning

How to suction your patient's mouth and trachea

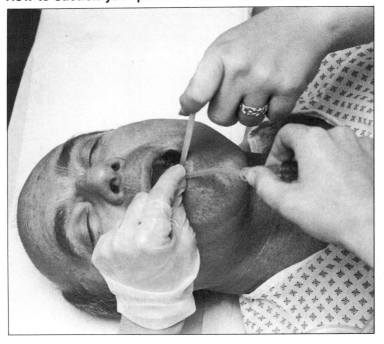

1 *Here's how to suction your patient orally:* First, ask another nurse to help you. Then, gather the equipment you'll need (including a tongue blade). For your own protection you may want to slip a sterile glove on one hand. When you open the patient's mouth, ask the other nurse to firmly depress the back of the patient's tongue. This will open his mouth wider (permitting you to see), move his tongue out of your way, and keep him from biting down on the catheter.

Now, suction his mouth as we show here, taking care to get along both sides of his tongue. If the patient also needs his trachea suctioned, replace catheter and glove before you proceed. Otherwise, you may introduce oral bacteria into his respiratory tract.

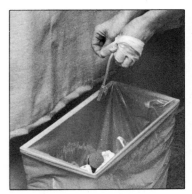

2 When you've completed the procedure, dispose of the contaminated catheter and glove in this manner: Use your ungloved hand to pull the glove inside out and over the catheter. Avoid touching either the outside of the glove or the catheter with your ungloved hand. Drop both into a wastebasket, as we show here.

How to suction your patient through an endotracheal or trach tube

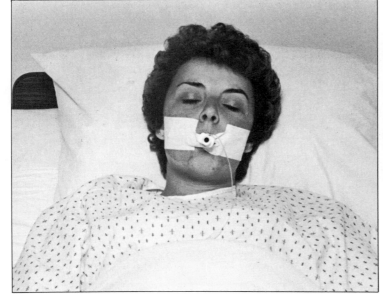

1 To properly suction your patient through an endotracheal or trach tube, start by assembling the necessary equipment, as explained on page 61. Then, disconnect the wide-bore humidified oxygen tubing attached to the patient's endotracheal or trach tube, and lay it across a towel on her chest. When you've completed these steps, use a hand-held ventilator with supplemental oxygen to hyperinflate the patient's lungs a few times before suctioning. (If she's already on a ventilator, see Section 4 of this Photobook for guidelines.)

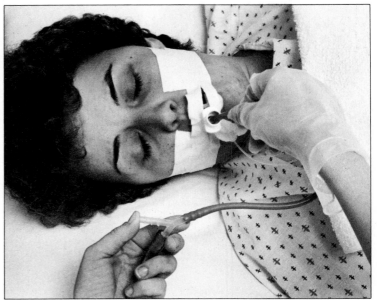

2 Now, gently insert the suction catheter into the patient's endotracheal or trach tube. Proceed with the suctioning procedure, as explained on page 60. After you've completed each insertion of catheter, hyperinflate the patient's lungs again with the hand-held ventilator. You may also need to suction around the mouth and outside of tube. Don't forget to reconnect the wide-bore oxygen tubing or ventilator.

Suctioning problems: How to solve and avoid them

Problem	Here's what to do	To avoid problem next time
You attempt to suction a patient and discover the equipment doesn't suction.	• Make sure unit is plugged in (if it's electric). • Make sure the unit is securely attached to wall socket. • Check for a tight fit on vacuum bottle lid. • Make sure tubing and catheter connections aren't loose. • Check switch to make sure it's on. • Make sure catheter isn't kinked.	• Check equipment carefully at the beginning of each shift. • Draw some sterile water or saline solution through the suction catheter to check it before you insert the catheter into the patient.
Patient goes into bronchospasm while you're suctioning him, and you're unable to remove catheter with gentle tugging.	• Don't use force to remove it. • Disconnect catheter from the connecting tubing, and let it act as an airway. • If bronchospasm doesn't subside immediately, give the patient oxygen by placing oxygen tube to catheter end and increasing prescribed liter flow. • When bronchospasm does subside, quickly remove catheter, and give patient prescribed amount of oxygen. Reassure him.	• Suction patient only when necessary. If possible, get him to cough up secretions. • Explain the procedure before you begin, to help patient relax. • Suction gently. • If the patient's having difficulty, remove the catheter before he has a bronchospasm and give him oxygen.
Your patient sounds congested, but you're unable to suction any secretions from his endotracheal tube or trach tube. Or, the secretions you *do* suction are extremely dry or viscous.	• Using a syringe (with the needle removed), instill 2 to 3 ml saline solution into the endotracheal tube or trach tube. • Hyperinflate the patient's lungs with a hand-held ventilator. • Proceed with suctioning. • Repeat procedure again later, if necessary, but only after you've given patient a chance to rest.	• Keep patient well hydrated. • Administer humidification therapy and aerosol treatments, as ordered. Or request an order from the doctor. • Don't give milk or milk products to a patient with tracheostomy, because they can thicken and increase sputum.
You're suctioning the mouth of an aphasic stroke patient and find that he won't cooperate with you.	• Try to calm him by speaking calmly and soothingly. • Ask another nurse to keep patient's mouth open with a padded tongue blade. This will keep him from biting down on the catheter.	• Regularly turn the patient from side to side so secretions will drain from his mouth naturally. • Encourage him to cough up secretions by demonstrating what you want him to do.
You're suctioning a patient through his nose and suddenly observe that his heart rate's dropped to 40.	• Stop suctioning immediately. • Remove catheter and give oxygen. • Monitor and document vital signs. • Notify doctor, if necessary.	• Avoid nasal suctioning unless other methods of removing secretions fail. • Closely observe patient's heart rate throughout the entire procedure.
You begin suctioning your patient and notice pink-tinged mucus.	• Check for signs of pulmonary edema. • Find out if he's been taking Isuprel, which can cause pink-tinged mucus. • Ask if he's just eaten red gelatin. • If none of these have occurred, perhaps you've injured the patient's trachea by suctioning him too vigorously.	• Keep your patient well hydrated so his mucosa won't get dry and be prone to injury. • Make sure catheter is correct size. Try a smaller size to minimize trauma. • Review the technique you're using to make sure it's correct.

Suctioning

Getting a sputum culture

Does your patient need a sputum culture? That's something for the doctor to decide, but you can help by watching for—and documenting—the following danger signs:
• unusual drainage around a tracheostomy site
• change in color, odor, quantity, or viscosity of the patient's sputum

• fever, malaise, tachycardia (late signs).

If the doctor orders a culture, use these guidelines to help you collect a sputum specimen that can be accurately analyzed by the laboratory:
• Collect the specimen first thing in the morning, if possible, because that's when the patient will be the most productive.

Have the patient brush his teeth and rinse his mouth before coughing into sputum cup.
• Because the specimen must originate from the lungs, make sure the patient coughs deeply enough. If you're using a suction catheter, make sure it extends all the way to the bronchus.
• Collect at least 5 cc to get an accurate analysis.

• If the patient has a contagious disease like tuberculosis, collect the sputum specimen in a nonporous container and label it "contaminated."
• Take the specimen to the lab immediately. Remember, sputum collection cups do not contain preservative.

Using a Lukin's trap

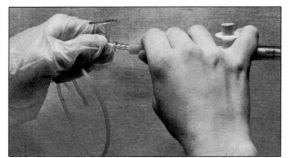

1 *If the doctor wants you to collect a sputum specimen from your patient for a laboratory analysis, you'll probably use a Lukin's trap like this one.* So before you begin suctioning your patient, you must hook up the trap between the catheter and the tube connecting it to the suction equipment. To do this, insert the trap's male adapter into the suction tubing, as shown.

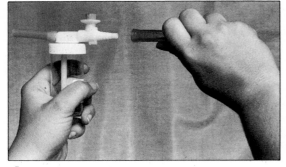

2 Next, slip on a sterile glove. With your gloved hand, insert catheter into the rubber tubing, as shown in this photo. Be sure cork on top of trap is secure. As you hold the catheter, allow trap to rest upright against your palm or wrist. Measure catheter to the correct size, and dip it in sterile water or saline to lubricate it. Be careful not to use too much, or it might be suctioned into the trap.

Now, suction patient according to the usual procedure, shown on page 64. *Nursing tip:* If the suction catheter you're using has no control valve, remove cork from the trap and control suction there or pinch catheter.

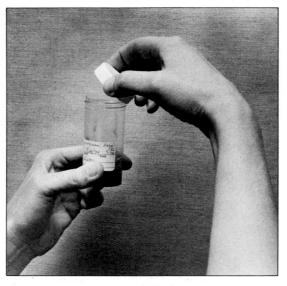

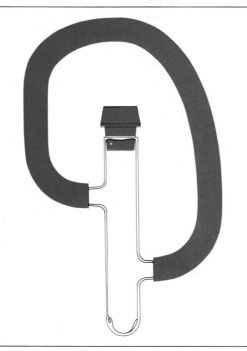

3 After you've finished suctioning, disconnect the Lukin's trap. Seal it with the extra cap that came with the trap. Take care not to touch the inside of the trap. Then, send the specimen to the lab as soon as possible.

4 You may be using a trap designed like this one. If you are, take care to keep it upright when you suction. To seal this type to send to the lab, connect the rubber tubing, as shown in this photo.

Emergency airway management

You may not always have an artificial airway or hand ventilator available when your patient needs emergency airway management or resuscitation. To help you cope in such an event, these pages show you:
• how to assess the quality of your patient's respirations and airway patency without a stethoscope or spirometer
• how to clear an obstructed airway without suction equipment
• how to ventilate the patient with or without a mechanical ventilator
• how to cope with special problems that occur during artificial respiration; for example, how to give mouth-to-stoma resuscitation
• how to determine the need for cardiopulmonary resuscitation.

MINI-ASSESSMENT

Does your patient have an obstructed airway?
Suspect airway obstruction when your patient:
• begins clutching at his throat
• suddenly loses the ability to speak
• displays exaggerated chest movements.
    To determine whether air is entering or leaving his lungs, cup your hand over the patient's nose and mouth to feel for exhaled air. Or place your ear close to his nose and mouth to listen for a rush of air while you watch for chest movement.
    Is your patient heading for a respiratory crisis? Know the signs of impending airway obstruction:
• wheezing; stridor
• exaggerated chest movements, especially during inspiration
• tachycardia
• changes in skin color: cyanosis or pallor
• restlessness, agitation, fearful facial expression.
    As you know, aspirated food or foreign objects are responsible for many cases of airway obstruction. Other causes include:
• unconsciousness, causing the tongue to fall back and block the airway
• severe trauma to face, neck, or upper chest
• acute tracheal edema from smoke inhalation or from face and neck burns.
    Remember, absence of breathing doesn't always mean the patient has an airway obstruction. He may have:
• cardiopulmonary arrest
• toxic effect from anesthetic or other drug
• respiratory paralysis from a neuromuscular disease like myasthenia gravis
• head or cervical spinal cord injury
• overoxygenation.
    Regardless of the cause, he needs immediate treatment.

Giving mouth-to-mouth resuscitation

1 *Sooner or later, you'll probably have to administer artificial respiration to restore someone's breathing. Such an emergency situation can occur outside the hospital or while you're on the job, as we've dramatized here. Here's how to cope with it.*
    Suppose you discover a patient lying on the corridor floor. First, determine whether or not he's unconscious by *gently* shaking his shoulder and asking him if he's O.K. If he doesn't respond, call for help immediately. *Caution:* Be careful when you shake such a patient, so you don't compound any injuries he may have.

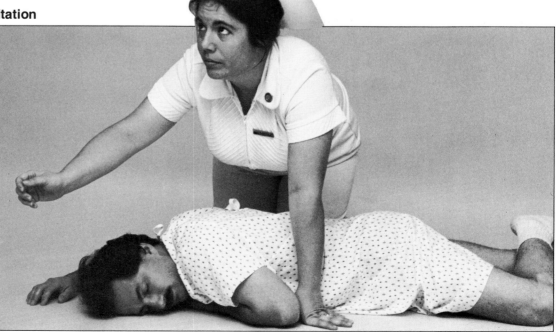

Emergency airway management

Giving mouth-to-mouth resuscitation continued

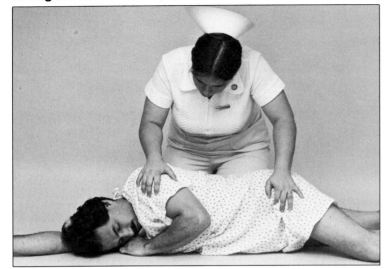

2 If the patient's lying face down, you must roll him over before you can administer the artificial respiration or cardiopulmonary resuscitation he may need. Take care when you turn him. Roll his body as a *unit*, as shown in this photo. If you suspect that he has a neck injury, keep one hand on his neck to support it. *Never twist the patient's body.*

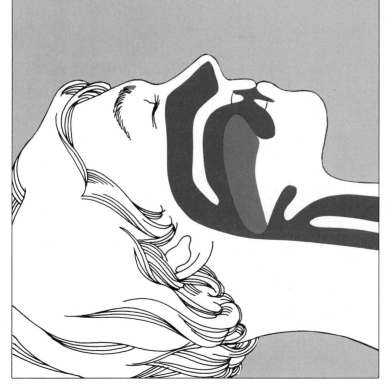

3 As soon as you have the patient lying flat on his back, make sure he has an open airway. When a patient's unconscious and in a supine position, the relaxed muscles in his lower jaw will allow his tongue to fall back and occlude his airway, as we've shown in this photo.

4 To open the patient's airway, gently hyperextend his neck by placing one hand beneath his neck (close to the back of his head) and the other hand on his forehead. Never hyperextend a patient's neck in this way if you think he may have a neck injury. Instead, use the modified jaw thrust, as shown on page 70.

Note: In some cases, hyperextending the patient's neck as we show here isn't enough to lift his tongue and open his airway. If it isn't, support his lower jaw by lifting his chin. (See caption 6.)

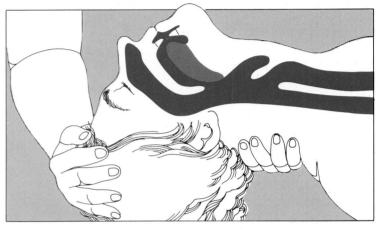

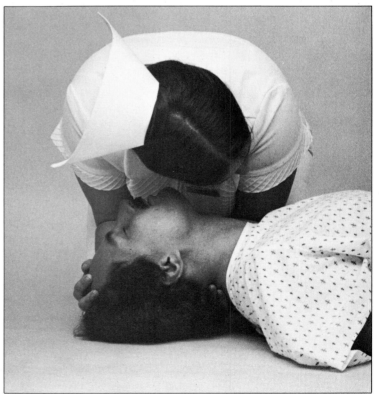

5 Now, check to see if the patient's breathing by placing your ear over his mouth and nose, and looking at his chest and abdomen. Listen and feel for air escaping during exhalation. Watch his chest to see if it rises and falls.

6 In some cases, hyperextending the patient's neck as we explained in Photo 4 isn't enough to lift his tongue and open his airway. If it isn't, support his lower jaw by lifting his chin. To do this, place your fingers under the boney (not soft) part of the lower jaw and bring his chin forward. Use your thumb to lightly depress the patient's lower lip; never use it to lift his chin.

If the patient has loose dentures, you'll find this method helpful for keeping them in place. However, take care not to lift and support the lower jaw so firmly that you completely close the patient's mouth.

Remove loose dentures if they're still a problem. Once again, listen and feel for breathing.

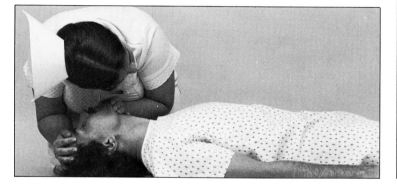

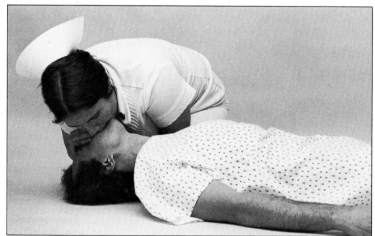

7 By now, your patient should have an open airway, which, in many cases, is enough to restore his breathing. If you notice that he's making respiratory efforts but you don't feel or hear air, check again for an obstructed airway. You'll find other ways to clear an obstructed airway on page 73.

Suppose you've opened the patient's airway, but he's still not breathing. Immediately begin artificial respiration (rescue breathing). To do this properly, use the hand you've place on his forehead to pinch his nostrils closed. Keep his head hyperextended, or his chin lifted with your other hand. Now, take a deep breath, open your mouth very wide and place it around the outside of your patient's mouth. Make a tight seal. Quickly blow four full breaths into the patient's lungs, without allowing time for them to deflate between breaths.

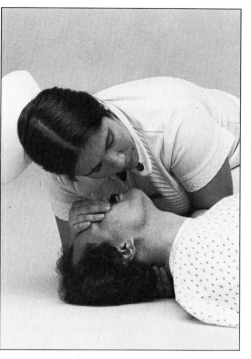

8 Turn your head and watch for his chest to fall as he exhales. If your efforts aren't ventilating the patient, make sure you're opening your mouth wide enough to get a tight seal.

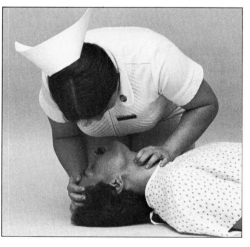

9 Now, feel for the patient's carotid pulse. To do this, place your fingertips on his trachea and slide them toward you, gently pressing on the *soft* part of his neck. Don't press down too hard or you may impair his airway.

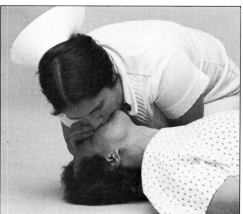

10 Suppose the patient's still not breathing, but you feel a pulse. Deliver one breath as described above, every 5 seconds. Recheck the pulse every 12 ventilations to make sure it's still present until breathing is restored. If no pulse is present, give immediate CPR.*

*Find out how to give CPR in the NURSING PHOTOBOOK *Dealing with Emergencies.*

Emergency airway management

Using the modified jaw thrust

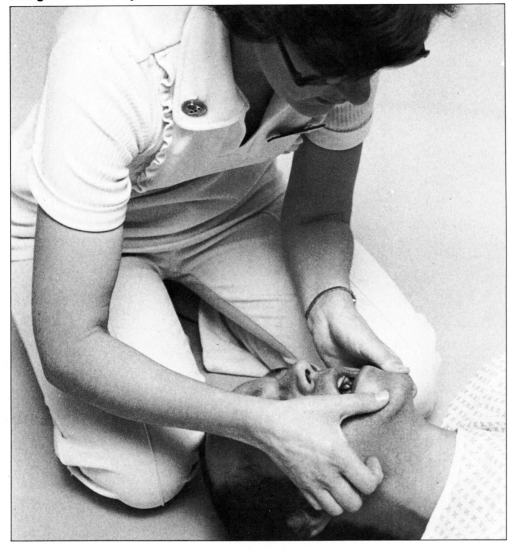

1 *Do you suspect neck injuries in a patient who obviously needs immediate artificial respiration? If you do, don't hyperextend his neck. Prevent further neck injuries by using the modified jaw thrust to open his airway.*

Here's how: First, kneel just behind the patient, as shown in this photo. Next, grasp the angles of his lower jaw with both hands and lift it forward. Properly done, this maneuver will tilt his head backward without hyperextending his neck. Retract the patient's lower lips to open his mouth.

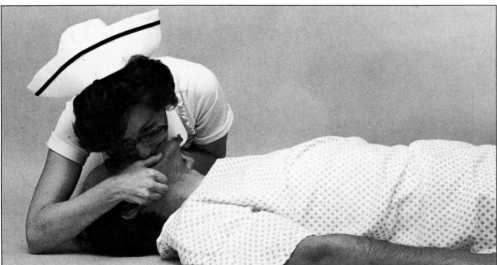

2 Maintain the modified jaw thrust as you deliver four quick breaths in succession, without waiting for the patient's lungs to deflate between breaths. Check for a carotid pulse to determine if he requires immediate cardiopulmonary resuscitation (CPR). If a pulse is present but he's still not breathing, continue to deliver one breath every 5 seconds until breathing's restored. Continue checking for a carotid pulse after every 12 breaths.

Giving artificial respiration to an infant

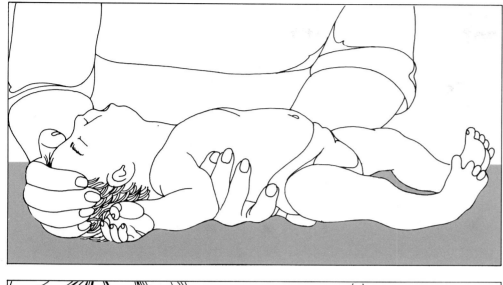

1 *When an infant needs immediate artificial respiration, you'll have to modify the basic procedure you'd use on an adult. Obviously, you'll still check for a possible airway obstruction and remove it, if you can. (For full details on how to do this, see page 73.)*

If no obstruction's present and the infant is still not breathing, perform the usual procedure for mouth-to-mouth resuscitation, with the following important changes.

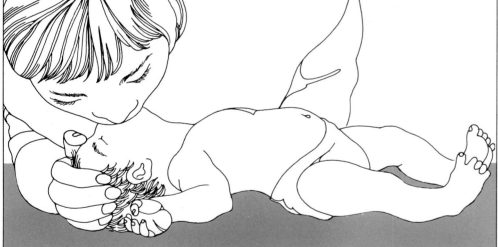

2 Don't hyperextend the infant's neck as much as you would an adult's. Doing so could seriously damage his spinal cord.

Ventilate the infant's lungs by sealing your mouth over both his mouth *and* nose.

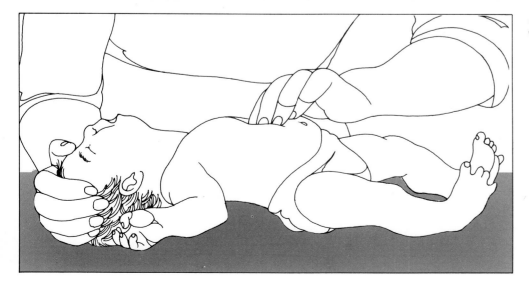

3 Administer only small breaths, like puffs of air, to inflate his lungs. Breathing that's more forceful than this could hurt him.

Watch for signs of gastric distention from artificial ventilation. If distention seems marked, relieve it by applying gentle pressure to the infant's upper epigastric region. Then, turn him on his side so he doesn't aspirate vomitus. Clear his airway quickly before you resume artificial respiration.

Emergency airway management

Mouth-to-nose resuscitation

If your patient's stopped breathing but he has facial injuries that prevent mouth-to-mouth resuscitation, give him mouth-to-nose resuscitation. You may also want to use this method if you can't get a tight seal over the patient's mouth because he has no teeth.

To do mouth-to-nose resuscitation properly, proceed as follows: First, hyperextend the patient's neck or use the modified jaw thrust to open his airway. Then, make sure the patient's lips are closed. Seal your mouth over his nose, pressing your cheek against his lips. Administer artificial respirations in the same way as described for mouth-to-mouth resuscitation. Don't forget to check for the patient's carotid pulse after the first four breaths and again after every 12 breaths. Start immediate cardiopulmonary resuscitation (CPR), if needed.

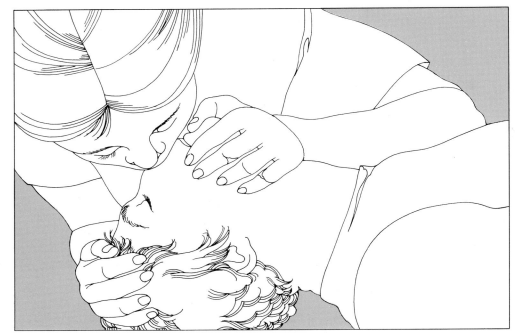

Mouth-to-stoma resuscitation

In some cases, you won't be able to administer mouth-to-mouth resuscitation to a patient who requires artificial respiration. If, for example, she has a neck stoma, you'll have to blow air into her lungs through her stoma. Air that's blown through her nose or mouth may not go past her trachea.

To give artificial respirations mouth-to-stoma, follow these instructions: First, make sure the patient's neck is flat. You don't have to hyperextend it to get an open airway. Now, cover her mouth and nose with one hand, as shown in this photo.

Seal your mouth over her stoma, and deliver four quick breaths in succession, without waiting for her lungs to deflate between breaths. Watch for the patient's chest to rise and fall. Remove your mouth from her stoma, and check the carotid pulse. If pulse is present, continue to administer one breath every 5 seconds until breathing's restored. If no pulse is present, give immediate CPR. *Important:* Always check for a carotid pulse after every 12 breaths, even if it was present when you started artificial respiration.

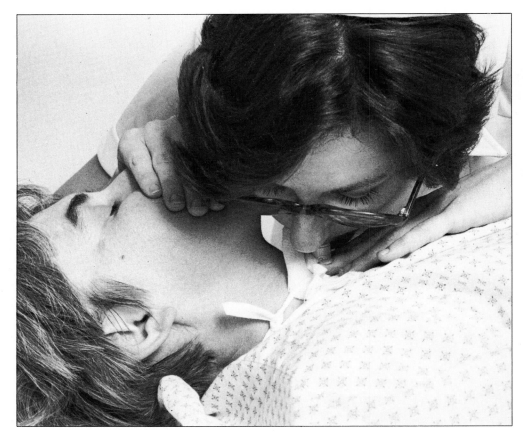

Dealing with airway obstruction

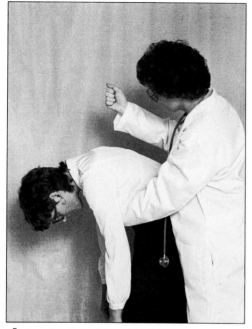

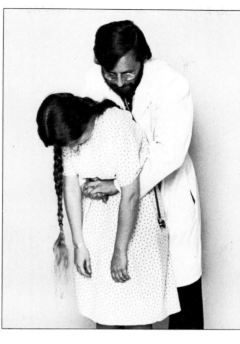

1 *Is a foreign object blocking your patient's airway? Quickly assess whether the obstruction's partial or complete. With partial obstruction, the patient may still have enough air exchange to allow forceful coughing. If he does, don't interfere with his efforts to expel the foreign object. But if the patient has poor air exchange, you'll need to intervene promptly. You'll recognize him by his weak, ineffective cough; stridor during inhalation (a crowing noise); extreme breathing difficulty; and possibly cyanosis. Treat such a patient as if his airway were completely obstructed.*

Remember, with complete obstruction, anoxia will cause death in approximately 3 to 5 minutes—unless breathing's restored. Try to relieve the obstruction by using these techniques:

Back blows. If the patient's standing or sitting down, get behind her, as shown in this photo. With the heel of your hand, deliver four sharp blows over her spine, between the scapulae. Place your other hand on her chest for support. If possible, position her head lower than her shoulders to maximize gravity's effect.

If the patient's lying down, kneel, and roll her onto her side, so she's facing you. Brace your thigh against her chest, and deliver four sharp blows to her back, as described above.

If the patient's a small child, hold him upside down as you deliver the back blows. *Caution:* Do this only in case of *complete* obstruction. If the patient's an infant, invert him over your arm.

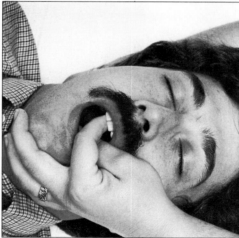

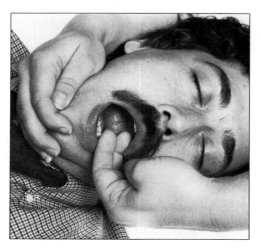

2 *Abdominal thrust.* Like back blows, abdominal thrusts produce a sudden increase in pressure in the patient's lungs and airways that may dislodge an upper airway obstruction. *For best results, use a combination of both techniques.* Here's how to perform the abdominal thrust:

If the patient's standing or sitting down, get behind her and wrap your arms around her waist. Place your fist with the thumb side against the patient's abdomen, above the navel but *below* the xiphoid process. Then, grasp your fist with your other hand and press it into the patient's abdomen with a quick upward thrust. Repeat four times.

If the patient's collapsed or you can't lift him, logroll him onto his back, and turn his head to one side. Kneel astride or alongside his hips, and place your hands, one on top of the other, over his epigastrium. Keep your shoulders directly over his abdomen. Now, with the heel of your bottom hand, press upward with a quick thrust. Repeat four times.

3 *Finger probe.* If the patient's unconscious and you strongly suspect an airway obstruction, immediately open his mouth using the crossed-finger technique. To do this properly, place your thumb on his lower teeth and your index finger on his upper teeth at the corner of his mouth. Force downward with your thumb and upward with your index finger.

4 Now, insert the index finger of your other hand deeply into the patient's throat, to the base of his tongue. Using a hooking motion, try to dislodge the foreign body and lift it out. Be careful not to force the object deeper into the airway. If you can't dislodge the obstruction, use back blows and abdominal thrusts.

To clear the mouth of vomitus, mucus, liquid, and foreign matter, use a sweeping motion with two fingers.

Once you've cleared the patient's airway, restore breathing with artificial respiration, if necessary.

Emergency airway management

In an emergency: How to use a hand-held resuscitator

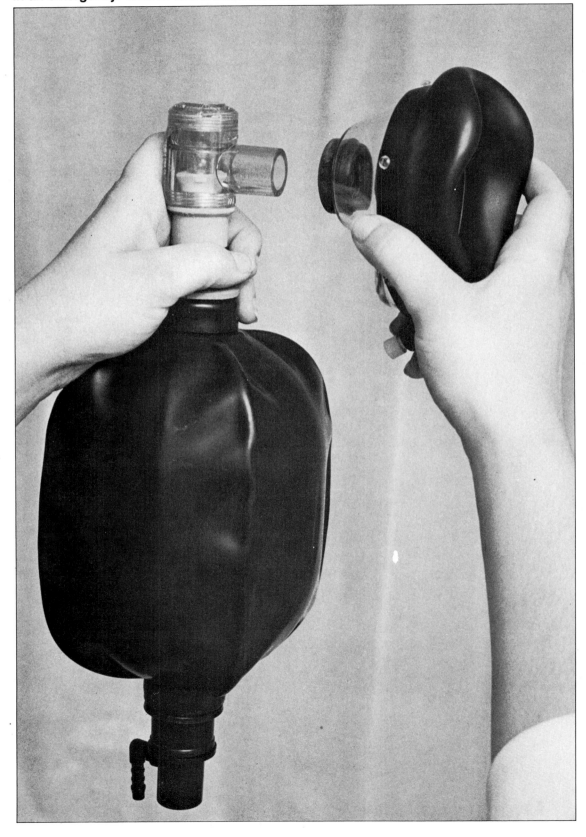

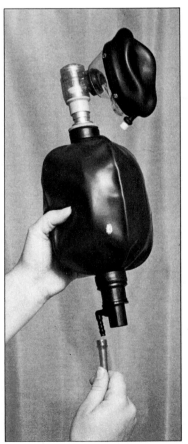

1 *Chances are, you won't have to administer mouth-to-mouth resuscitation long in an emergency situation like the one we described on page 67. In a hospital or clinic, someone will arrive momentarily with a hand-held resuscitator.*

One familiar brand is the Narco Air-Shields AMBU® Re-suscitator. Here's how to use it.

First, attach the mask to the bag, as shown in this photo. You're now ready to ventilate the patient.

2 When time permits, connect the resuscitator to the oxygen wall unit. Attach one end of the tube to the bottom of the bag and the other end to the nipple adapter on the flowmeter. You may want to add an oxygen reservoir bag to the resuscitator, if one is available.

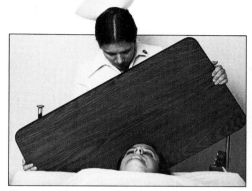

3 Make sure you have an adequate working area. To insure this, remove the bed's headboard, if possible, and pull the bed away from the wall. Then, step between the bed and the wall with the resuscitator.

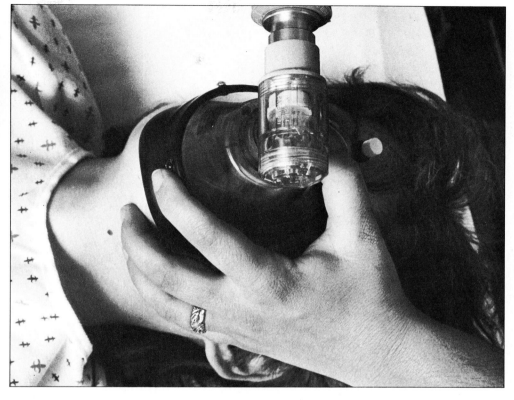

4 Hyperextend the patient's neck, if it isn't already, and place the triangular-shaped mask over his face. To do this correctly, make sure the apex of the triangle is over the bridge of his nose and the base is between his lower lip and chin. Place your fingers and thumb as shown in this photo, to hold the mask in place. Exert firm pressure to keep the neck hyperextended and the mask sealed tightly.

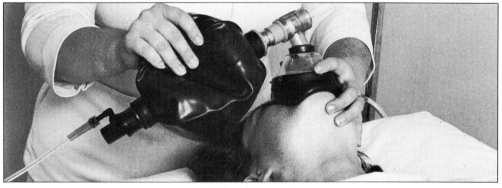

5 Now, with the other hand, compress the bag, as shown, every 5 seconds for an adult. With each compression you're delivering approximately 1 liter of air.

If you're ventilating an infant's lungs, you'll use a smaller size resuscitator and compress the bag once every 3 seconds.

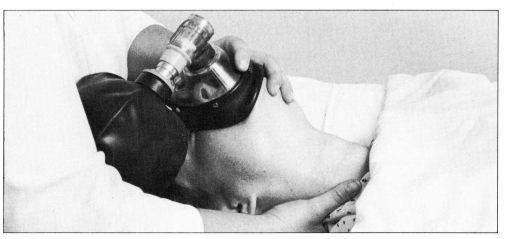

6 If you have small hands and need both of them to hold the mask in place, keep the patient's neck hyperextended. Then, position yourself as shown in this photo, and use the lower part of your arm to compress the bag against your side. Watch for the patient's chest to rise and fall each time you compress the bag. If it doesn't, check the mask. Chances are, it's not sealed tightly enough. Attempt to correct the problem by repositioning your hands.

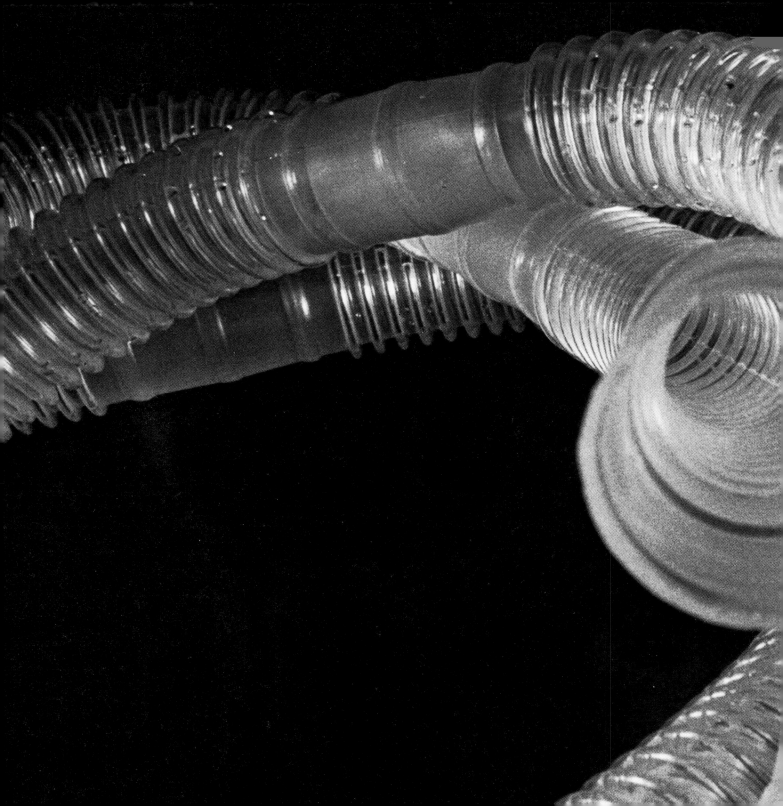

Giving Oxygen and Humidification

Blood gases
Oxygen equipment
Humidifiers and nebulizers
Oxygen delivery systems
Patient positioning

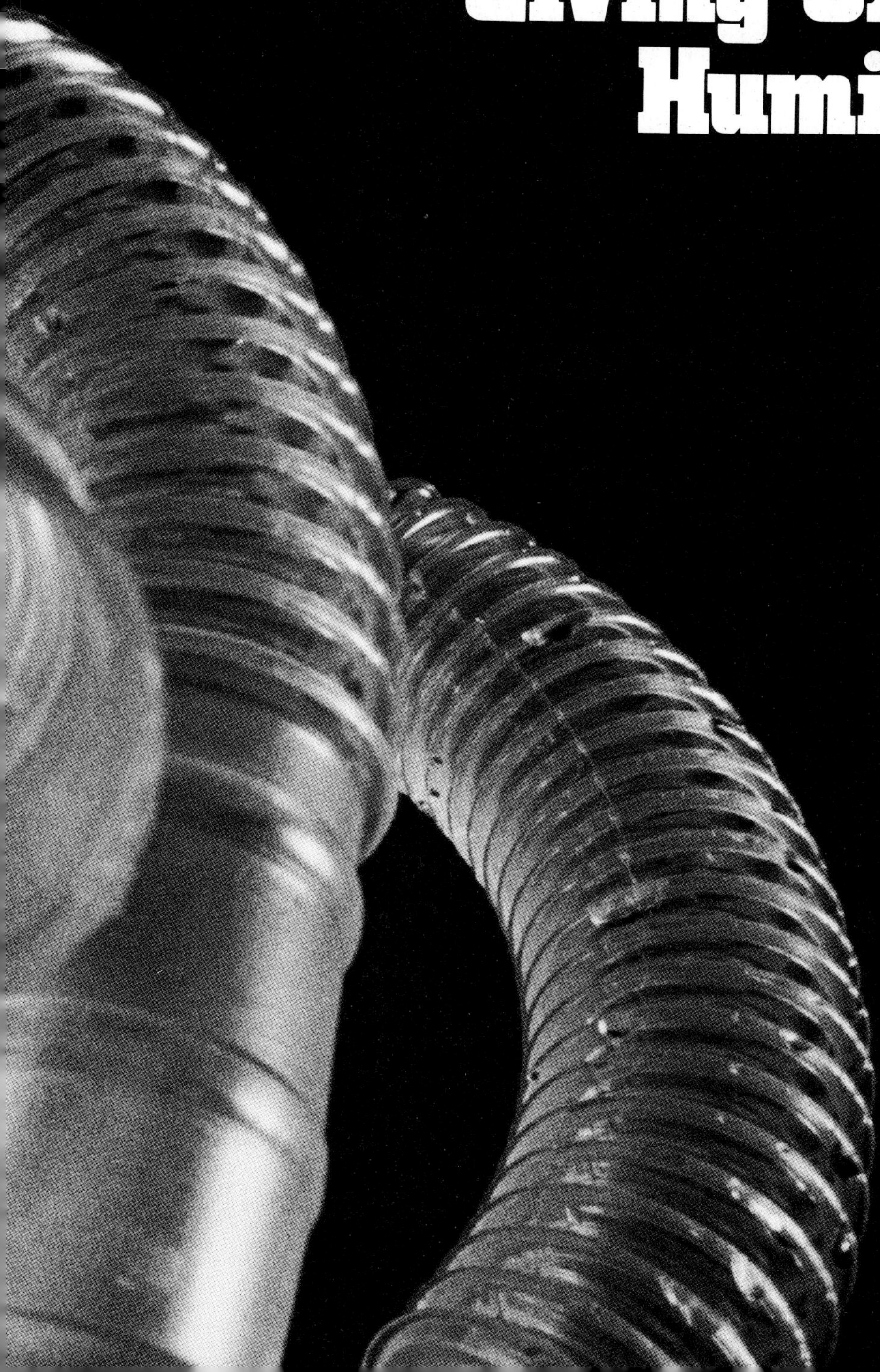

Blood gases

How well is your patient meeting his oxygen needs? Arterial blood gas studies can help to answer this, as well as other vital questions about his condition.

But do you know how to draw an arterial blood sample for laboratory evaluation? Specifically, how do you heparinize a syringe? Perform the Allen's test? Choose the correct needle angle?

If you need the answers to these and other questions nurses ask about blood gas studies, study the photostories on these pages. In them, you'll find step-by-step instructions for drawing an adequate arterial blood sample, and helpful nursing tips that'll make the job easier.

MINI-ASSESSMENT

The Allen's test: How to do it

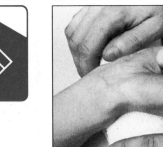

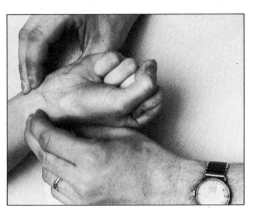

1 *Planning to draw blood from the radial artery? Before you do, use the Allen's test to see if the patient gets enough blood through her ulnar artery to supply her hand in case of occlusion. Here's how to do it:*

First, have the patient rest her arm on the bedside table. Support her wrist with a rolled towel. Ask her to clench her fist.

2 Now, use your index and middle fingers to exert pressure over both the radial and the ulnar arteries. *Hold for a few seconds.*

3 Without removing your fingers, ask the patient to unclench her fist. You'll notice her palm is blanched because you've impaired the normal blood flow with your fingers.

4 Now, release pressure only over the patient's ulnar artery. Note whether her hand becomes flushed, which indicates the rush of oxygenated blood to the hand. If it does, you can safely proceed with the radial artery puncture. If it doesn't, repeat the test on the other arm. If neither arm produces a positive result, choose another site for the puncture. (For other arterial sites, see the chart on page 82.)

How to draw blood from a radial artery

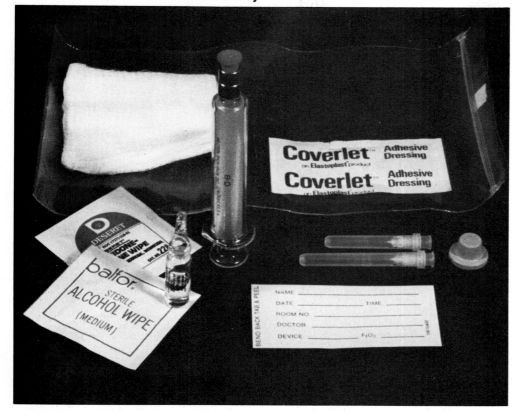

1 To do this procedure correctly, you'll need: 10 ml glass syringe, I ml aqueous heparin (1:1000), Luer-Lok cap or small cork, ½" needle (23G), 1½" needle (20G), Betadine solution, alcohol swabs, 4" x 4" gauze pad, 1" adhesive dressing or tape, and an iced specimen bag with label.

2 Before entering the patient's room, always heparinize the syringe to help prevent the specimen from clotting on its way to the lab. Here's how: First, wash your hands thoroughly. Then, attach a 20-gauge needle to the syringe. Break open the ampule and draw 1 ml of heparin into the syringe. Pull the plunger back past the 7 ml mark, rotating the barrel as you do. Now, hold the syringe in an upright position as shown in the photo opposite. Then, slowly force the heparin toward the hub of the syringe as you continue to rotate the barrel. Stop when you still have at least 0.1 ml heparin in the syringe.

[Inset] Heparinize the needle, too. To do this, remove the first needle and replace it with the 23-gauge needle. Continue to hold the syringe upright, but tilt it slightly. Now, push the plunger all the way up to eject the remaining heparin. Tilting the syringe keeps heparin from running down the sides of the needle where it can come in contact with the patient's skin and possibly irritate it. Cap the needle.

Blood gases

How to draw blood from a radial artery continued

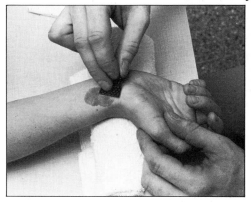

3 Now, you're ready to draw blood from the patient's artery. Before you do, take time to prepare him. First, tell him what you're going to do. Then, have him rest his arm on the bedside table and support his wrist with a rolled towel. *Important:* If you haven't performed the Allen's test yet, do so now (see page 78). If the test's positive, clean the area around the radial artery with a Betadine swab, as shown, using a circular motion.

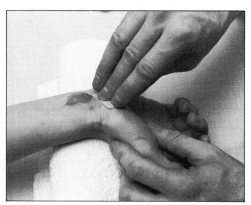

4 Wipe the Betadine off with an alcohol swab. If you don't, the sticky solution may hinder your efforts to palpate the artery.

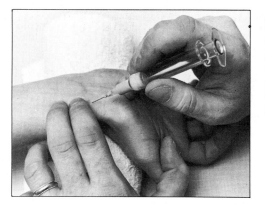

5 With your first two fingers slightly apart, palpate the radial artery. As soon as you locate a strong pulse, release the pressure, but don't move your fingers. Now, as we show in this photo, hold the needle at a 45° angle over the radial artery, with the bevel up. Take care not to touch the needle or you'll contaminate it.

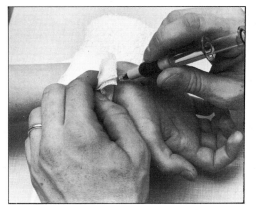

6 Without changing the needle angle, carefully puncture the skin. You'll know when the needle enters the artery, because blood will spontaneously fill the syringe. Draw 3 to 5 ml of blood for an adequate specimen. If the syringe doesn't fill immediately, you may have pushed it all the way through the artery. Pull needle back slightly. If you still don't get a specimen, withdraw needle completely and start over with a fresh heparinized needle. Never make more than two attempts to draw blood from one site. Instead, try another site. Withdraw needle and apply pressure over artery with sterile gauze pad.

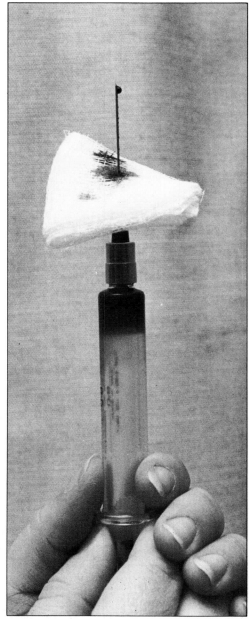

7 *Important:* Is there an air bubble in the syringe? You'll have to remove it, or it'll affect the oxygen level of the blood gas measurements. Call another nurse to apply pressure to the patient's artery. Then try to remove the bubble by holding the syringe upright and tapping it lightly with your finger. If the bubble doesn't disappear, hold the syringe upright and pierce a 2" x 2" gauze pad or alcohol swab with the needle, as shown. By slowly forcing some of the blood out of the syringe, you'll eliminate the air bubble. The gauze pad will catch the blood that's wasted.

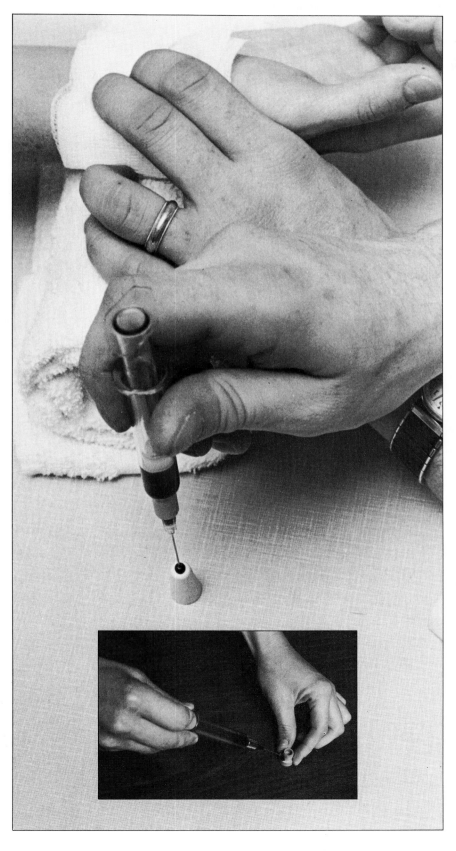

8 In any case, be sure to have the syringe cork and iced specimen bag (labeled) nearby. As you continue to apply pressure, use your free hand to insert the needle into the cork.

[Inset] If you can't find the cork or none was included in the prepackaged kit, substitute a stopper from a Vacutainer test tube. To do this, get someone else to maintain firm pressure on the patient's artery. Then, as we show in this photo, stick the end of the needle into the stopper at an angle, to avoid the stopper's hollow center.

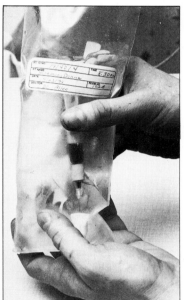

9 Slide the capped or corked syringe into the labeled specimen bag, and send it to the lab. If you don't have an iced bag, place the syringe in a Styrofoam cup of ice water.

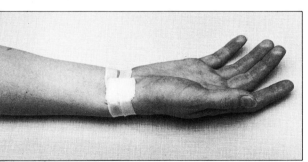

10 Apply pressure to the radial injection site for at least 5 minutes. If the patient has an abnormally long clotting time or is taking anticoagulants, you may need to apply pressure longer. Finally, apply a tight bandage over the puncture site, as shown in this photo, using two strips of tape. To do so, hold the gauze pad in place and attach one end of the tape to the dorsal side of the patient's wrist. Pull the tape toward the pad, exerting enough tension to create a small skin fold, and attach the other end securely. Never wrap tape completely around the wrist or you may impair the patient's circulation.

Apply the second strip in the same way. When you are done, the patient's arm will look like this.

Blood gases

Drawing arterial blood: Sites and angles

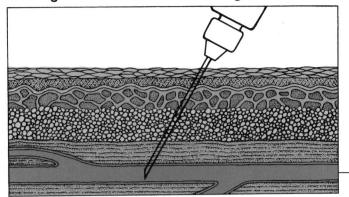

Puncture site: Brachial artery
Needle angle: 60° angle, to match the location of artery at that site
Advantage: Higher arterial blood pressure than at radial site, though not as great as at femoral site
Nursing tip: Apply pressure to site for 7 to 10 minutes.

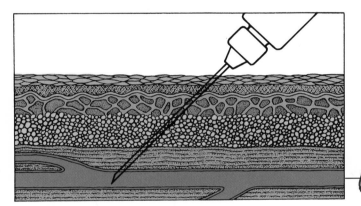

Puncture site: Radial artery
Needle angle: 45° angle, so entire bevel of the needle's inside the artery
Advantage: Most accessible, with fewest potential complications
Nursing tip: Apply pressure to site for at least 5 minutes.

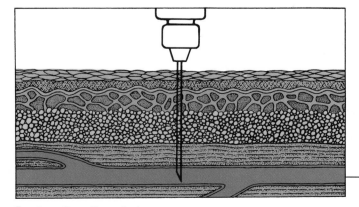

Puncture site: Femoral artery
Needle angle: 90° angle, to avoid abdominal cavity and nearby nerves
Advantage: Highest arterial blood pressure; commonly chosen in cases of cardiac arrest
Nursing tip: Apply pressure to site for at least 10 minutes.

Drawing blood from an arterial line

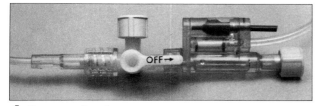

1 *If your patient has an arterial line with a stopcock valve like the one here, do the following to draw an arterial blood sample for lab evaluation:*

First, get a 5 ml disposable syringe, a 5 ml heparinized glass syringe with cap, a towel or disposable drape, and an iced specimen bag with label. If you're not sure how to heparinize a syringe, see page 79.

Now, examine this photo carefully. As you can see, the three-way stopcock lets you either deliver I.V. fluid to the patient or draw arterial blood, depending on which way you turn the stopcock handle.

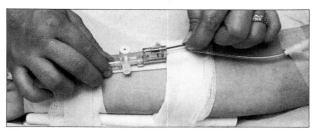

2 Before drawing arterial blood, turn the stopcock handle so it points up toward the syringe port. Place a towel or disposable drape under the patient's arm to protect the bedding. If you use a sterile drape, you can place the syringe cap on it later.

Now, as we show in this photo, gently pull the pigtail to flush the arterial line. As you do so, you should see an increased flow rate in the I.V. line's drip chamber. If you don't, suspect a line obstruction. *Important:* Don't continue the procedure until you've determined the problem's cause and corrected it.

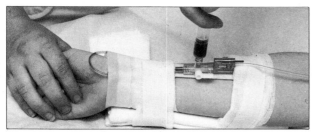

3 Next, unscrew the stopcock cap and attach the 5 ml disposable syringe. If the syringe is a Luer-Tip, simply push it into place. If it's a Luer-Lok, turn the barrel clockwise and secure it. Once the syringe is in place, turn the stopcock handle back toward the pigtail, which'll allow you to draw blood into the syringe. Draw off 5 ml of blood. Then, turn the stopcock handle so it's straight up again. Remove the filled syringe and discard it. Why? Because some of the first blood you've drawn was probably trapped in the I.V. line and won't be suitable for an accurate blood gas analysis.

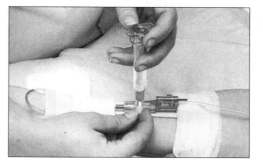

4 When you've completed these steps, attach the heparinized glass syringe to the syringe port, as shown in this photo.

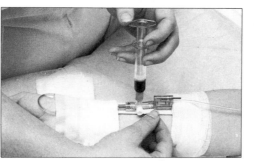

5 Turn the stopcock handle back toward the pigtail. This time arterial pressure will force blood into the syringe spontaneously. Draw 3 to 5 ml, depending on your laboratory's requirements.

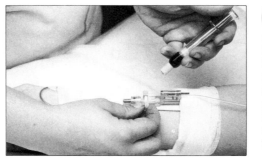

6 Turn the stopcock handle straight up again and remove the syringe. Be careful to hold the barrel as well as the plunger of the syringe, or it may come apart and spill the sample. Cap the syringe and put it into the iced specimen bag. Write the necessary information on the label, and send the bag to the lab immediately.

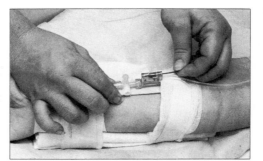

7 Remember to flush the line after you've drawn the blood. Then flush the syringe port. To do this, first turn the stopcock handle so it points away from the pigtail, as shown in this photo. Gently pull the pigtail, allowing I.V. fluid to clear blood from the syringe port.

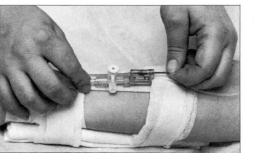

8 Replace the cap on the syringe port. Then, turn the handle so it's pointing straight up again. Pull the pigtail once more to completely flush the line.

Blood gases

Understanding arterial blood gas measurements

Here's an easy way to interpret your patient's arterial blood gas (ABG) measurements. But, before looking at these graphs, review the normal values chart on the next page.

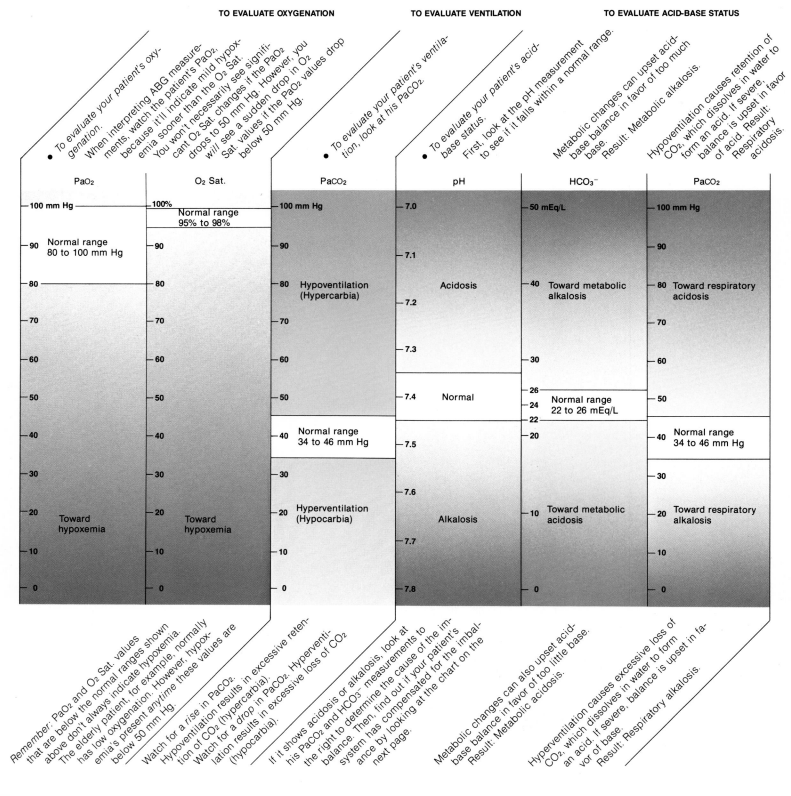

TO EVALUATE OXYGENATION

• *To evaluate your patient's oxygenation.*
When interpreting ABG measurements, watch the patient's PaO_2, because it'll indicate mild hypoxemia sooner than the O_2 Sat. You won't necessarily see significant O_2 Sat. changes if the PaO_2 drops to 50 mm Hg. However, you will see a sudden drop in O_2 Sat. values if the PaO_2 values drop below 50 mm Hg.

TO EVALUATE VENTILATION

• *To evaluate your patient's ventilation, look at his $PaCO_2$.*

TO EVALUATE ACID-BASE STATUS

• *To evaluate your patient's acid-base status.*
First, look at the pH measurement to see if it falls within a normal range.

Metabolic changes can upset acid-base balance in favor of too much base. Result: Metabolic alkalosis.

Hypoventilation causes retention of CO_2, which dissolves in water to form an acid. If severe, balance is upset in favor of acid. Result: Respiratory acidosis.

PaO₂	O₂ Sat.	PaCO₂	pH	HCO₃⁻	PaCO₂
— 100 mm Hg	—100%	— 100 mm Hg	— 7.0	— 50 mEq/L	— 100 mm Hg
	Normal range 95% to 98%				
— 90 Normal range 80 to 100 mm Hg	— 90	— 90	— 7.1	— 90	
— 80	— 80	— 80 Hypoventilation (Hypercarbia)	— 7.2 Acidosis	— 40 Toward metabolic alkalosis	— 80 Toward respiratory acidosis
— 70	— 70	— 70	— 7.3	— 30	— 70
— 60	— 60	— 60			— 60
— 50	— 50	— 50	— 7.4 Normal	— 26 / 24 Normal range 22 to 26 mEq/L / 22	— 50
— 40	— 40	— 40 Normal range 34 to 46 mm Hg	— 7.5	— 20	— 40 Normal range 34 to 46 mm Hg
— 30	— 30	— 30			— 30
— 20 Toward hypoxemia	— 20 Toward hypoxemia	— 20 Hyperventilation (Hypocarbia)	— 7.6 Alkalosis	— 10 Toward metabolic acidosis	— 20 Toward respiratory alkalosis
			— 7.7		
— 10	— 10	— 10			— 10
— 0	— 0	— 0	— 7.8	— 0	— 0

Remember: PaO₂ and O₂ Sat. values that are below the normal ranges shown above don't always indicate hypoxemia. The elderly patient, for example, normally has low oxygenation. However, hypoxemia's present anytime these values are below 50 mm Hg.

Watch for a *rise* in PaCO₂. Hypoventilation results in excessive retention of CO₂ (hypercarbia). Watch for a *drop* in PaCO₂. Hyperventilation results in excessive loss of CO₂ (hypocarbia).

If it shows acidosis or alkalosis, look at his PaCO₂ and HCO₃⁻ measurements to the right to determine the cause of the imbalance. Then, find out if your patient's system has compensated for the imbalance by looking at the chart on the next page.

Metabolic changes can also upset acid-base balance in favor of too little base. Result: Metabolic acidosis.

Hyperventilation causes excessive loss of CO₂, which dissolves in water to form an acid. If severe, balance is upset in favor of base. Result: Respiratory alkalosis.

Has your patient's system compensated for this imbalance? To find out, look at the *other* blood gas measurement; for example, if your patient's *primary* imbalance is from an abnormal PaCO₂ level, look at the HCO₃⁻ level.

Use these charts to help:

ALKALOSIS

Cause

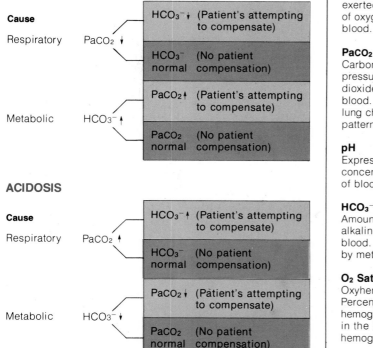

Respiratory   PaCO₂ ↓
- HCO₃⁻ ↓ (Patient's attempting to compensate)
- HCO₃⁻ normal (No patient compensation)

Metabolic   HCO₃⁻ ↑
- PaCO₂ ↑ (Patient's attempting to compensate)
- PaCO₂ normal (No patient compensation)

ACIDOSIS

Cause

Respiratory   PaCO₂ ↑
- HCO₃⁻ ↑ (Patient's attempting to compensate)
- HCO₃⁻ normal (No patient compensation)

Metabolic   HCO₃⁻ ↓
- PaCO₂ ↓ (Patient's attempting to compensate)
- PaCO₂ normal (No patient compensation)

Normal arterial blood gas values

Arterial blood gas (ABG)	Normal values
PaO₂ Oxygen tension. Partial pressure exerted by the small amount of oxygen dissolved in arterial blood.	80 to 100 mm Hg
PaCO₂ Carbon dioxide tension. Partial pressure exerted by carbon dioxide dissolved in arterial blood. Primarily influenced by lung changes and respiratory pattern.	34 to 46 mm Hg
pH Expression of hydrogen ion concentration. Clinical measure of blood acidity.	7.34 to 7.45
HCO₃⁻ Amount of bicarbonate or alkaline substance dissolved in blood. Primarily influenced by metabolic changes.	22 to 26 mEq/L
O₂ Sat. (SaO₂) Oxyhemoglobin saturation. Percentage of oxygen carried by hemoglobin. Most of the oxygen in the blood is carried by hemoglobin.	95% to 98%

How to fill out an ABG requisition slip

The following patient information is needed to correctly interpret ABG measurements. Make sure it's *current* when you include it on the requisition slip.
- rectal temperature
- respiratory rate
- room air or oxygen. If the patient's receiving oxygen, give the flow rate.
- FIO₂ and tidal volume, if patient's on a ventilator.

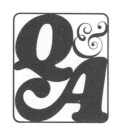

Drawing arterial blood for blood gas measurements: Some special tips

About to draw arterial blood to get blood gas measurements? Here are the answers to some questions you'll probably ask:
- *Should you numb the area with a local anesthetic like xylocaine?* No, for several reasons. First, it will delay the procedure unnecessarily. Second, the patient may have an allergic reaction to the drug. Third, the vasoconstriction produced by the drug may keep you from doing a successful puncture.
- *How can you help the patient who's afraid of needles?* Prepare the needle and ice out of his sight. Speak softly and calmly, reassuring him as much as possible. Take extra time locating the artery so you're successful with the first puncture.
- *Should you turn off any oxygen the patient's receiving?* No, unless ordered. But you must check the patient's chart to make sure he's been getting the prescribed oxygen concentration for at least 15 minutes before you draw the blood. Indicate the liter flow on the slip you send to the lab. If no oxygen's in use, simply indicate that the patient's breathing room air (21% oxygen).

- *If the patient's just had an IPPB treatment, how long must you wait before drawing arterial blood?* Approximately 20 minutes. Any less could alter the blood gas measurement.
- *Suppose the patient has a bleeding disorder or is taking anticoagulants?* Take special precautions to prevent excess bleeding. After you draw the blood, apply pressure to the puncture site for 5 to 10 minutes longer than usual. Don't worry about the heparin you used to prepare the syringe. It can't affect the patient's clotting time, because it wasn't injected into his bloodstream.
- *Can medications alter the patient's blood gas measurements?* Yes, but only the patient's PCO₂ level. Some of the drugs that may increase PCO₂ level are bicarbonates, hydrocortisones, chronically used laxatives, thiazides, and viomycin sulfate (Viocin). Some of the drugs that may decrease the patient's PCO₂ level are tetracycline, nitrofurazone (Furacin*), methicillin (Staphcillin*), and acetazolamide (Diamox*).

Oxygen equipment

Perhaps you're not aware of all the ways you can give a patient oxygen. For example, you may be familiar with wall units, but not cylinders. To review the correct ways to use both portable and stationary supplies of oxygen, study the photostories on the following pages.

Setting up oxygen equipment

1 If your hospital doesn't have a wall unit, you'll probably use one of the larger cylinders (size G or H) for oxygen delivery. To set up the cylinder, first unscrew the cap to expose the handle or knob.

[Inset A] Next, connect the flowmeter and regulator to the cylinder outlet valve. To do this, fasten the regulator nut to the threaded connector on the cylinder.

[Inset B] Use a wrench to tighten the connection. In most cases, you'll find the wrench strapped to the cylinder. Attach the humidification bottle.

[Inset C] Next, crack the cylinder to clear any dust from the line. To do this, slowly turn the handle or knob counterclockwise until you hear a loud rush of air. Then quickly turn the knob clockwise to shut off the gas. Always crack a cylinder *before* you enter your patient's room; otherwise, the loud noise may frighten him. In some hospitals, you may be instructed to crack the cylinder *before* you attach the flowmeter. This may keep dust particles from getting into the regulator.

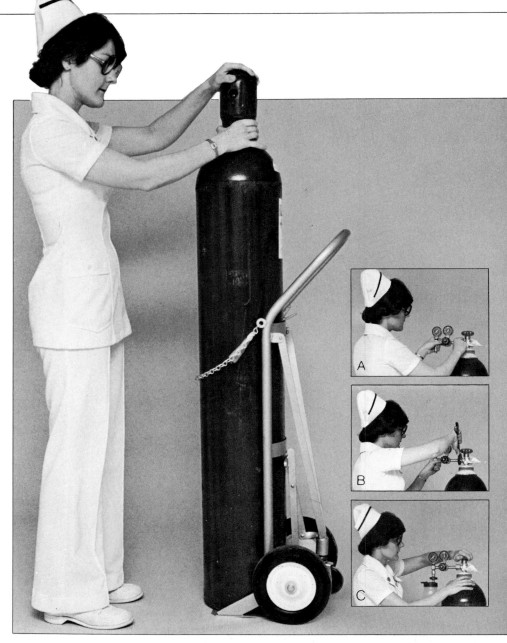

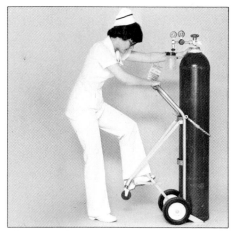

2 To transport the cylinder in its carrier, raise the third wheel, as shown, and snap it into place.

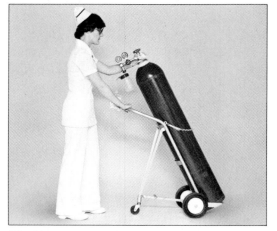

3 Move the cylinder to the patient's room. For safety, keep the chain securely attached as long as it's in the carrier.

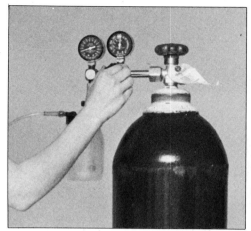

4 When the cylinder's in place, release the lock on the third wheel and stand it upright. Adjust the liter flow. To do this, turn the valve directly under the regulator gauge, which is on the right. To increase the flow, turn clockwise; to decrease it, turn counterclockwise. The gauge on the left is the flowmeter, which indicates oxygen flow in liters per minute.

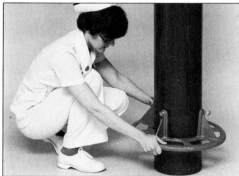

5 Suppose you want to remove the carrier and leave the cylinder standing by itself. In that case, make sure you slip a metal skirt over the cylinder before you attach the humidification bottle. Avoid striking the gauges and connector when you do so. Then, position the skirt flat on the floor and tighten the bolts.

6 If your patient can walk or he's being moved in a wheelchair or stretcher, you'll probably need to set up a small cylinder. Here's how to do it: First, locate the three holes on the cylinder stem, as shown in the photo.

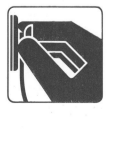

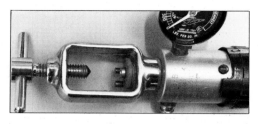

7 Next, examine the yoke attachment. You'll see three pegs, which correspond to the holes on the cylinder stem.

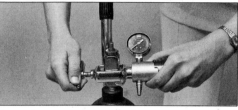

8 Now, holding the yoke attachment firmly in both hands, make sure the pegs are correctly seated in the proper holes. Turn the viselike screw on the side of the yoke attachment to secure it.

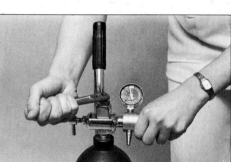

9 Crack the cylinder by fitting a wrench over the stem and turning it counterclockwise until you hear a loud rush of air. Then, quickly turn it back clockwise to shut off the gas.

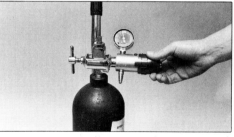

10 Next, adjust the liter flow by turning the dial on the right. Turning the dial clockwise increases the flow; turning it counterclockwise decreases it. *Note:* This particular model yoke does not have a flowmeter.

MINI-ASSESSMENT

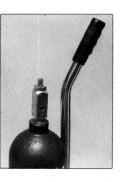

How to transport a patient who's receiving oxygen
Suppose you're caring for a patient who's getting oxygen. Before you transport him to another unit of the hospital for X-rays or treatments, consider these guidelines:
• *Is he too sick to transport?* A portable X-ray, or bedside treatment may be necessary.
• *Can he be moved without oxygen?* If he's breathing comfortably and continuous oxygen is not ordered, send him without it. However, make sure oxygen's available at his destination in case he'll need it.
• *Does he become overly anxious without oxygen?* Send a portable oxygen cylinder with him.
• *Does he need a semi-Fowler's or high-Fowler's position to breathe?* If so, he'll need a stretcher that can be adjusted to the necessary position. Use pillows, if necessary. Remind the health-care professionals at his destination about his requirements.

Oxygen equipment

Behind the wall unit

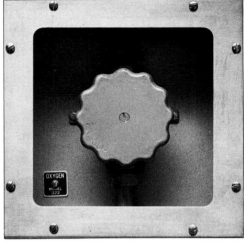

Where does the oxygen you use come from? You may use a cylinder, but in most large hospitals, you'll rely on a wall unit. The oxygen that flows through these wall units comes from huge liquid oxygen storage tanks (9,300 gallons or larger) located in the hospital's engineering department.

Because the ratio of liquid oxygen to oxygen gas is 1 to 860, a standard liquid oxygen tank will supply almost 26 million liters of gas. However, if the tank runs out, a bank of oxygen cylinders, or manifold, will automatically begin operation.

The oxygen pressure in most wall units is standardized—and controlled in the engineering department—at 50 pounds per square inch (50 psi). By adjusting the flowmeter, you control the oxygen flow delivered to the patient in liters per minute.

Important: In case of fire, immediately shut off the oxygen supply to your floor by turning the main valve. Know where this valve is located on your floor.

Using a duplex adapter

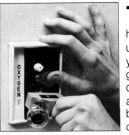

1 Use a duplex adapter if: You have only one wall unit for oxygen and you must give oxygen to two patients; or if you have to alternate a patient between two types of oxygen therapy.

To use the duplex adapter, lift the protector on the wall outlet, as shown here, and push the adapter straight in. Listen for a clicking sound to tell you it's locked into the valve.

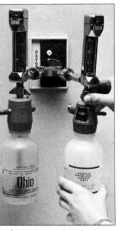

2 Then, attach both flowmeters to the duplex adapter in the same way you attached the adapter to the wall outlet valve. (Make sure they're turned off before you do.) Then, press with a slight clockwise twisting motion to insure a firm fit. Connect other attachments, such as bubble bottles, to each flowmeter before you slowly open the flowmeter valve. As oxygen flows into the flowmeter, the ball float will rise. *Note:* You don't have to run both flowmeters simultaneously for the duplex adapter to work. One part of the adapter can be empty. And, of course, each flowmeter has its own shut-off valve.

Teaching your patient how to use oxygen at home

Does the doctor want your COPD patient to continue his oxygen therapy at home? If so, you'll want to prepare him, and make sure he understands the precautions. Demonstrate the following: how to attach a flowmeter and regulator, how to crack an oxygen cylinder, and how to use a humidifier.

How can you be sure your patient has grasped what you've told him? First, keep your instructions simple. Avoid medical jargon; use familiar terms. Then, ask him to repeat the demonstration to clear up any difficulties he may have. Be sure to document what you've done in the patient's discharge summary.

To help him remember your instructions after he returns home, give him a patient teaching card like the one below. Include the family in the discussion.

Dear Patient:
To help you breathe more easily, your doctor wants you to continue using oxygen at home. You can buy or rent the equipment you'll need at the following medical supply company: _____

When you order it, specify that you want a cylinder of *medical oxygen*, not the industrial type. If the doctor says it's okay for you to move around a lot, you may want to consider a portable unit.

Always keep at least a 3-day supply of oxygen on hand. If you decide on oxygen with a continuous electrical source, talk to your supplier about getting a small emergency tank to use in case of power failure.

Important: Although oxygen by itself is not combustible, it'll feed a fire if one occurs. Be careful. Don't use around a stove or gas space heater. Don't smoke or light matches around the cylinder when oxygen's in use. Post a *No Smoking* sign, and call it to the attention of visitors.

Keep the water in the humidifier at the correct level, and don't let it run dry. Adjust the cylinder's flowmeter exactly as the doctor ordered and *don't change it.* If you notice increased trouble breathing, call your doctor immediately.

Also notify him at once in any of these situations:
• if you feel unusually restless or upset
• if your breathing gets irregular
• if you feel abnormally drowsy
• if your lips or fingernail beds look blue
• if you have trouble concentrating or get confused.

Don't assume more oxygen will make you feel better or breathe more easily. Get in touch with the doctor, or go to the hospital's emergency department.

When you give oxygen

• *Do* secure each cylinder in its proper skirt, even when it's in storage. This will keep it from tipping over and discourage staff members from dragging or sliding it, which may produce friction.
• *Do* make sure the regulating·device and flowmeter are working properly.
• *Do* crack the cylinder before you enter the patient's room, to avoid scaring him. When you crack a cylinder, always point the outlet valve away from yourself and others.
• *Do* open the pressure valve slowly.
• *Don't* store cylinder at a temperature above 125° F. (51.7° C.).
• *Don't* cover cylinder with bed linen or clothing. This may cause a dangerous rise in temperature. It'll also keep you from monitoring the liter flow gauge easily.
• *Don't* allow combustible materials, such as oil, grease, or alcohol, near cylinders, wall valves, gauges, or fittings. Although oxygen itself isn't combustible, it'll feed a fire if one occurs.
• *Don't* permit smoking in the patient's room. Instruct visitors accordingly.
• *Don't* wear clothing made from wool, silk, or synthetic fabrics. The static electricity produced by these fabrics might generate a spark that could ignite a fire.
• *Do* post a warning sign stating that oxygen's in use. Explain necessary precautions to the patient, his family, and other visitors.
• *Do* keep all valves closed when oxygen's not in use, even on cylinders that register empty.

Humidifiers and nebulizers

As you know, the air a person breathes is normally warmed and humidified as it travels through the nasopharyngeal airway on its way to the lungs. Suppose, however, that your patient's nasal airway is obstructed; or that he has an endotracheal or tracheostomy tube; or that he's receiving a high concentration of oxygen. Under any of these conditions he won't be getting enough humidity in the air he breathes. As a result, secretions thicken and collect, narrow his airways, and impair his breathing.

How can you help? To compensate for the lack of humidity reaching his lower respiratory tract, you need to supplement the air's moisture content. To do this, you'll use either a humidifier or a nebulizer. The difference between these two kinds of devices is that humidifiers deliver water vapor, whereas nebulizers deliver a mist of water droplets. Many humidifiers and nebulizers have heating elements to raise the moisture's temperature up to 140° F. (60° C.). To find out exactly how to use the various types of humidifiers and nebulizers, read the following pages thoroughly.

Using an aerosol face mask

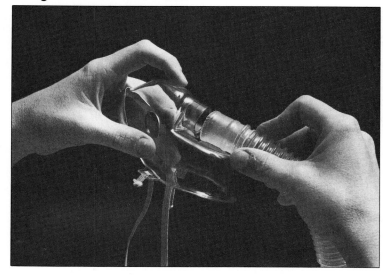

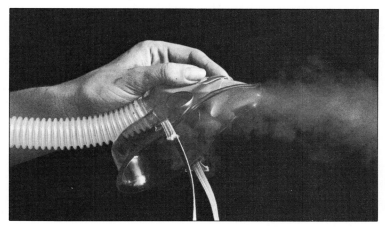

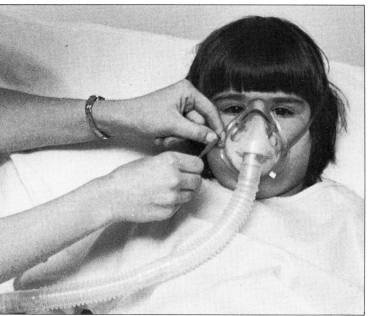

1 Suppose you're caring for a child with respiratory difficulty. The doctor may order an aerosol face mask to deliver humidified air or oxygen. Why? Because a child will tolerate a mask better than a nasal cannula or nasal catheter. Besides the aerosol face mask, you'll also need wide-bore tubing, a nebulizer *to provide humidification,* a flowmeter, and compressed air or oxygen. Your hospital may stock nebulizers with built-in heating elements. If not, and you're going to give warm humidity, you'll need a separate heating element.

Begin by connecting the flowmeter to the compressed air or oxygen source. Then, fill the nebulizer with sterile water, and attach it to the flowmeter. Attach one end of the wide-bore tubing to the chimney on the aerosol face mask, as shown here. Next, attach the other end of the tubing to the nebulizer.

2 Turn on the flowmeter until you *see* a mist. To create an adequate mist, you'll need a flow of 10 to 12 liters per minute. Check the tubing for leaks.

3 Place the mask over the child's nose and mouth. Next, slip the elastic strap around the back of her head, and position it above her ears. Adjust the metal strip over her nose by pinching it into shape. Then, gently pull the headstrap to tighten it, as shown here. Make sure the mask fits snugly, but not uncomfortably. Prevent pressure sores by placing 4'' x 4'' gauze pads under the strap. Keep the wide-bore tubing from kinking or twisting. *Nursing tip:* A semi-Fowler's, or Fowler's, position will give your patient's lungs more room to expand. However, before elevating the patient, make sure her condition doesn't require a supine position.

Humidifiers and nebulizers

Using the mini-nebulizer

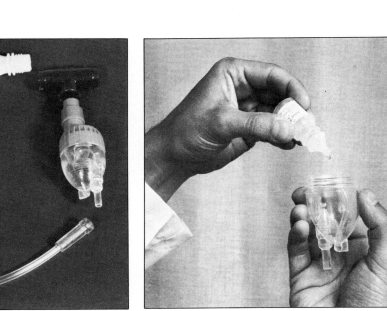

1 *Does the doctor want your patient to receive treatments with a mini-nebulizer? To help her use it properly, follow these patient-teaching guidelines:*

First, ask yourself: Is the patient unfamiliar with the mini-nebulizer treatments? Briefly explain how they'll help her, as you're preparing the kit for use. Inside the kit, you'll find oxygen connector tubing, a hand-held nebulizer cup with lid, a T-piece, and a mouthpiece. You'll also need a fresh bottle of sterile saline, as well as any medication the doctor's ordered. For dosage guidelines, see the Nurses' Guide to Aerosol Therapy Drugs on the opposite page.

2 Now, open the nebulizer's lid. Break open the bottle of sterile saline, and place the prescribed amount of liquid in the nebulizer. Add any medication the doctor may have ordered. Carefully replace the lid.
[Inset] Next, securely attach the T-piece to the nebulizer, as the nurse is doing in this photo.

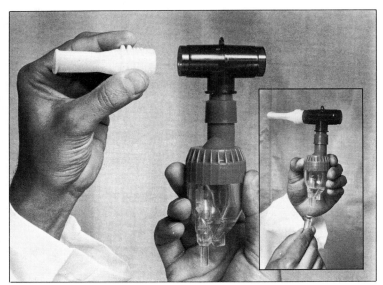

3 Then, hold the mouthpiece, as we show here, and insert it into the T-piece.
[Inset] Attach the connector tube to the unit delivering oxygen or compressed air. Then, connect it to the nebulizer, as you see here. Turn the flow rate up to 10 liters per minute, or until you observe an adequate mist coming from the mouthpiece.

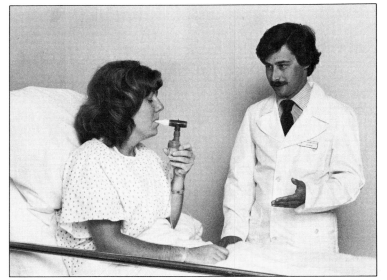

4 Now, instruct the patient to sit up as straight as possible for maximum chest expansion. Tell her to hold the nebulizer upright and to close her lips around the mouthpiece. Then, ask her to inhale deeply and hold for several seconds before exhaling. Watch to make sure she's following instructions correctly. If possible, remain with her for the time it takes to complete the treatment. Finally, document how well the patient tolerated the treatment. Be specific; include any signs of the medication's effects.

Nurses' guide to aerosol therapy drugs

Drug	Indications and dosages	Side effects	Nursing considerations
epinephrine 1:1000 Adrenalin, Medihaler-Epi*, Primatene Mist, Vaponefrin	*For use as a bronchodilator:* **Adults:** 0.2 mg per dose. One to two inhalations, as needed. Do not administer more than three inhalation treatments per day.	Blood pressure changes, tachycardia, excitement, tremor. May also cause angina when coronary insufficiency is present.	• Monitor vital signs closely. • Don't use if solution is brown or contains precipitate. • Tell patient to wait 1 to 2 minutes between inhalations. • Have patient rinse mouth after each treatment to prevent oropharynx dryness. • Don't use concurrently with isoproterenol, although you may give these two drugs alternately.
isoproterenol hydrochloride Isuprel*, Medihaler-Iso*	*For use as a bronchodilator:* **Adults:** 0.5 ml of 1:200 solution in 2 to 2.5 ml normal saline inhaled over 15 minutes. One to two inhalations four to six times daily. Do not administer more than six inhalations per day.	Hypotension, tachycardia, nausea, headache, flushing, palpitations; parotid swelling (with prolonged use).	• Monitor vital signs closely. • Don't use if solution is brown or contains precipitate. • Don't give concurrently with epinephrine. • Have patient rinse mouth after each treatment. Instruct him not to swallow medicine or rinse water. • Tell patient that sputum and saliva may be pink for a while after inhalation.
isoetharine Bronkometer, Bronkosol	*For use as a bronchodilator:* **Adults:** 0.25 ml to 1 ml diluted 1:3 with saline and administered IPPB over 10 to 15 minutes once every 4 hours. When given with hand nebulizer, three to seven inhalations undiluted every 4 hours. When given with aerosol nebulizer, one to two inhalations, as needed.	Blood pressure changes, palpitations, nausea, tachycardia.	• Monitor vital signs closely. • Don't give concurrently with epinephrine. • Tell patient using aerosol nebulizer to wait 1 minute after first dose before repeating.
metaproterenol sulfate Alupent*, Metaprel	*For use as a bronchodilator:* **Adults and children (over age 12):** Two to three inhalations every 3 to 4 hours, as needed. Do not administer more than 12 inhalations per day.	Nervousness, weakness, drowsiness, tremor, tachycardia, hypertension, palpitations, vomiting, nausea, bad taste; possible cardiac arrest (with excessive use).	• Use with extreme caution in patients with hypertension, coronary artery disease, hyperthyroidism, or diabetes. • Teach patient how to use metered-dose unit. (For tips, see patient instruction card and photostory on page 94.) • Tell patient to call doctor if he does not respond to usual dose. • Protect drug from light.
acetylcysteine Airbron**, Mucomyst, NAC**	*For use as a mucolytic:* **Adults and children:** 1 to 2 ml of 10% to 20% solution by direct instillation into trachea. Or, 3 to 5 ml of 20% solution, inhaled three to four times daily. Or 6 to 10 ml of 10% solution, inhaled three to four times daily. In croupette: Up to 300 ml daily.	Rhinorrhea, hemoptysis, stomatitis, nausea, bronchospasm (mainly in asthmatics).	• Use with caution in asthmatics, elderly or debilitated patients. • Use nonreactive metal, plastic, or glass when you administer by nebulization. • Store drug in refrigerator after opening, and use within 96 hours. • Monitor and document cough (type and frequency). • Urge patient not to smoke. • Don't mix with antibiotics.
tyloxapol Alevaire	*For use as a mucolytic or as vehicle to deliver bronchodilators (isoproterenol, epinephrine, or phenylephrine):* **Adults:** 10 to 20 ml of 0.125% solution administered by IPPB, given over 30 to 90 minutes, three to four times daily. Or, 500 ml of 0.125% solution administered by continuous aerosol over 12 to 24 hours.	Nausea	• Incompatible with chlortetracycline. • When used as vehicle, add bronchodilators just before use. • Monitor and document cough (type and frequency). • Urge patient not to smoke.
beclomethasone dipropionate Vanceril*	*A corticosteroid used to treat bronchial asthma:* **Adults:** 100 mcg total given in two inhalations three to four times daily. Don't administer more than 20 inhalations daily. **Children (ages 6 thru 12):** One or two inhalations three to four times daily. Do not administer more than 10 inhalations daily.	Hoarseness, dry mouth. Death from adrenal insufficiency during and after transfer from systemic steroids to beclomethasone.	• Contraindicated as a primary treatment for status asthmaticus. • Check patient's mouth for signs of fungal infections. Send culture to lab, if necessary. • Instruct patient how to use inhaler properly.
dexamethasone sodium phosphate Decadron Respihaler*, Decadron Turbinaire*	*A corticosteroid used to treat bronchial asthma:* **Adults:** *Respihaler:* Three inhalations three to four times daily. Do not administer more than 12 inhalations daily. *Turbinaire:* Two sprays in each nostril two to three times daily. **Children:** *Respihaler:* Two inhalations three to four times daily. Do not administer more than eight inhalations daily.	Laryngeal or pharyngeal fungal infections, throat irritation, hoarseness, and coughing.	• Instruct patient how to use inhaler properly. • Check patient's mouth for signs of fungal infection. Send culture to lab, if necessary.
cromolyn sodium Aarane, Intal*	*Used in combination with other drugs to treat patients with bronchial asthma:* **Adults and children (over age 2):** 20 mg inhaled four times daily at regular intervals.	Bronchospasm, cough, nasal congestion, wheezing, angioedema, dizziness, dysuria, joint swelling, lacrimation, headache, nausea, rash, urticaria, swelling of parotid gland.	• Instruct patient how to use inhaler properly. • If improvement occurs, it'll occur within 4 weeks. • Discontinue drug if eosinophilic pneumonia occurs. • Not used for emergency treatment. • Sudden discontinuation of this drug may necessitate reintroduction of oral corticosteroids.

*Available both in the United States and Canada.
**Available only in Canada.

Humidifiers and nebulizers

Nurses' guide to humidifiers and nebulizers

Apparatus	Advantages	Disadvantages	To avoid complications
Cold bubble	• Can be used with all oxygen masks, nasal cannulas, and nasal catheters.	• Delivers only 20% to 40% humidity • Can't be used on patient with bypassed upper airway; for example, a tracheostomy.	• Replace humidifier, or refill it, as water evaporates. *Important:* Always empty the jar completely; then refill it to the proper level. • If it's not disposable, sterilize humidifier before using it for another patient.
Cascade, or bubble, humidifier (heated)	• Delivers 100% humidity at body temperature • Functions as mainstream humidifier with ventilator • Most effective of all evaporative humidifiers.	• Temperature control can become defective from constant use, causing device to over- or underheat. • If correct water level isn't maintained, patient's mucosa can become irritated from breathing hot, dry air.	• Check cascade temperature every 2 hours. Don't let it exceed 101.6° F. (38.6° C.). • Check the water level at least once every 4 hours. When you add water, empty the reservoir completely; then refill to correct level. • Attach reservoir tightly. • If humidifier is overheated, unplug it and let it cool. Attach another cascade to continue humidification of the patient.
Pneumatic (jet) reservoir nebulizer (heated or cool)	• Heated nebulizer provides 100% humidity; cool nebulizer provides 40% humidity. • Useful for long-term therapy • Can provide both oxygen and aerosol therapy • Attaches to wall unit or cylinders.	• Nondisposable units increase risk of bacterial growth. • Condensation can collect in wide-bore tubing. • If correct water level in reservoir isn't maintained, patient's mucosa can become irritated from breathing hot, dry air. • Infant can easily become overhydrated from mist.	• If patient's upper airway is bypassed, use a heated nebulizer. • Check water level in reservoir at least once every 4 hours. When you add water, empty the reservoir completely; then refill to correct level. • Drain condensation from wide-bore tubing as soon as it collects. Don't drain water back into reservoir. • Make sure the nebulizer's always delivering a visible mist. • Weigh infant daily. Watch for signs of overhydration: weight gain, pulmonary edema, rales, electrolyte imbalance.
Molecular humidifier (heated)	• Delivers 100% humidity at body temperature • Disposable, except for heating element • Newer kinds are totally disposable.	• Same as for cascade humidifier • Infant can easily become overhydrated from mist.	• Observe same precautions listed for cascade humidifier. • Change tubing filters every time you change tubing. Don't use same filter for more than one patient. • Check mist temperature near infant's mouth. Don't let it exceed 95° F. (35° C.) because humidification will be too great. • Weigh infant daily. Watch for signs of overhydration: weight gain, pulmonary edema, rales, electrolyte imbalance.

Nurses' guide to humidifiers and nebulizers continued

Apparatus	Advantages	Disadvantages	To avoid complications
Metered-dose nebulizer	• Effectively delivers bronchodilator; each spray delivers a measured amount of medication.	• Difficult to assemble • Patient may use it excessively, because it's available without a prescription.	• Instruct patient how to use nebulizer. Give him a patient teaching card like the one on page 94. • Make sure patient doesn't exceed prescribed daily dosage. • Put mouthpiece and cap on nebulizer after each use to prevent contamination.
Ultrasonic nebulizer	• Delivers 100% humidity • About 90% of the particles will reach the lower airways, where they're effective. • Loosens secretions.	• May precipitate bronchospasms in patient with asthma • Lacks built-in oxygen delivery system • Increased water absorption may cause overhydration, leading to pulmonary edema or increased cardiac work load.	• Closely observe patient during and immediately after therapy. His secretions may be so copious and thin that you'll have to assist him. • Watch for signs of overhydration: weight gain, pulmonary edema, rales, electrolyte imbalance.
Intermittent positive pressure breathing (IPPB)	• Mechanically dilates bronchi and lungs; delivers bronchodilator to patient who can't generate an adequate tidal volume • May prevent atelectasis • Counteracts pulmonary congestion or edema; helps clear bronchial secretions • Can give treatment with oxygen or compressed air, depending on doctor's order.	• Delivers only 40% to 50% oxygen • Some COPD patients can't tolerate IPPB treatments with oxygen; when this happens, use compressed air. • May decrease venous return.	• Encourage patient to take slow, deep breaths. Don't allow him to become tachypneic. • Avoid excess pressures and high flow rates. Monitor pulse rates before, during, and after treatment. Sudden increase could indicate reaction to bronchodilator. (See drug chart on page 91.) • Watch COPD patients for signs of carbon dioxide narcosis: for example, lethargy and decreased respiratory rate. • Patients with cardiac or pulmonary deficiencies may develop decreased venous return. • Don't use in patients with hemoptysis, pneumothorax, active TB, or subcutaneous emphysema. • Don't use immediately postop pneumonectomy or lobectomy. • Don't overdo treatments with saline solution, because they're not as effective as previously believed.
Maxi-mist or mini-nebulizer	• Conforms to patient's physiology, allowing him to inhale and exhale with his own power • Causes less air trapping than IPPB • Can be used with compressed air, oxygen, or compressor pump • Compact, disposable unit.	• Procedure can take a long time if patient requires the nurse's assistance. Patient must be alert and cooperative. Medication may not distribute evenly if patient doesn't breathe properly.	• Instruct the patient to breathe slowly and deeply. Take time to coach the weak or elderly patient. Assist by holding the apparatus, when necessary. • Instruct the patient to keep the medicine cup upright during treatment. • Make sure tubing connections are tight; check for a good mist.

Humidifiers and nebulizers

How to use a metered-dose nebulizer

Has the doctor prescribed metered-dose nebulizer therapy for your patient? Teach him how to use the nebulizer properly. Find a quiet place where you can show him the following step-by-step procedure. Tailor your teaching to his learning skills; give him the opportunity to ask questions. Don't demonstrate the nebulizer for him; have him go through the procedure by himself, while you explain each step. Then give him a copy of the following teaching aid.

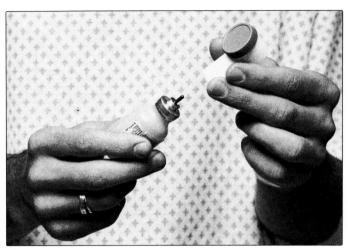

1 Dear Patient: The doctor wants you to use a metered-dose nebulizer at these times: _____ The medicine you'll inhale in the spray will help you breathe easier.

To get the most from this therapy, follow your doctor's orders exactly. These guidelines will help you use the metered-dose nebulizer correctly.

First, remove both the mouthpiece and its protective cap from the bottle as shown in this photo.

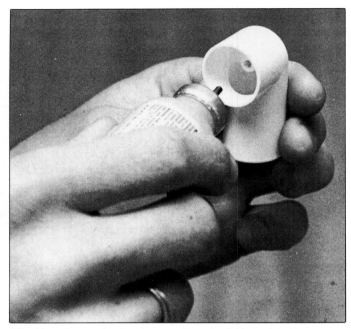

3 Now, insert the bottle stem into the hole inside the mouthpiece.

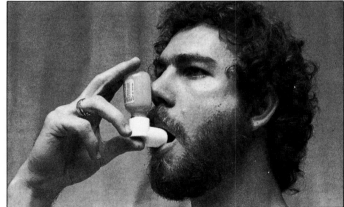

2 Then, carefully snap off the cap, and turn the mouthpiece sideways.

4 Next, invert the bottle and place the mouthpiece near your mouth. Exhale, pushing as much air as you can from your lungs. Then place the mouthpiece in your mouth and close your lips loosely around it. Inhale deeply as you press the bottle and mouthpiece together quickly. Release. Hold your breath for 3 to 5 seconds before exhaling. This will permit the medicine to penetrate and settle in your lungs.

Finally, wash the mouthpiece with clear water to prevent clogging.

Oxygen delivery systems

Did you know two kinds of oxygen delivery systems exist? High-flow and low-flow. Each type's capable of delivering both large and small concentrations of oxygen, yet, they differ. How?

Picture the typical low-flow apparatus: nasal catheter, nasal cannula, simple face mask, partial rebreather, or nonrebreathing mask. These devices let the patient inhale room air, which mixes freely with the oxygen. As the patient's ventilatory pattern changes, so does the concentration of oxygen he receives. Low-flow systems are economical and comfortable, but they don't give a fixed concentration of oxygen.

On the other hand, high-flow systems deliver a precise amount of oxygen, regardless of the patient's ventilatory patterns. Most of these systems utilize a venturi device that controls how much room air is entrained. The orifice size regulates the ratio of room air to oxygen, which in turn controls the oxygen's velocity, which directly affects the oxygen concentration. Changes in the patient's respiration don't affect the FIO2 as long as the correct liter flow's used. This section will tell you what types of high-flow and low-flow oxygen delivery systems are available, as well as their individual benefits.

MINI-ASSESSMENT

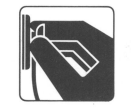

Does your patient need oxygen?

He may, if he has any of these problems when he arrives in your unit:

Decreased cardiac output; for example, from arrhythmias, myocardial infarction, hypovolemia, or increased vascular resistance

Decreased PaO2 in arterial blood gas measurement; for example, from bronchospasm, respiratory infection, COPD, drug overdose, or lobar atelectasis

Reduced oxygen-carrying capacity of blood; for example, from anemia, carbon monoxide poisoning, or methemoglobinemia

Increased need for oxygen; for example, from fever, burns, or hypothyroidism.

No matter what the patient's condition has been, stay alert for these changes that may indicate he now requires oxygen: restlessness, confusion, headache, nausea, tachypnea, dyspnea, decreased oxygen saturation, decreased PaO2 in arterial blood gas measurement, cardiac arrhythmias, tachycardia, or hypertension.

PRECAUTIONS

Oxygen therapy danger signs

Respiratory depression
When a patient has COPD, hypoxia becomes his main stimulus to breathe. If you give him too much oxygen, you may remove that stimulus and cause apnea. Prevent it by watching for these danger signs: somnulence and decreased respiration rate. Avoid giving high concentrations of oxygen. Make sure you have a mechanical ventilator handy in case of emergency.

Circulatory depression
When a patient has COPD, hypoxia can cause vasoconstriction. Oxygen therapy reverses this condition and dilates the blood vessels. It may also cause a serious drop in the patient's blood pressure. Prevent this by taking frequent CVP readings and monitoring his blood pressure for changes.

Atelectasis
When a patient receives a high oxygen concentration, the oxygen is exchanged, and the remaining nitrogen is washed from his lungs. This can lead to atelectasis. Do your best to prevent it by making sure your patient coughs and deep breathes on schedule. Hyperinflate his lungs, if necessary.

Oxygen toxicity,
When a patient receives a high oxygen concentration for a prolonged period, serious lung damage or blindness (in newborn infants) can occur. To prevent this, intervene to improve patient's ventilation with chest physiotherapy and suctioning. Monitor blood gas measurements for signs of improvement.

Oxygen delivery systems

Giving oxygen through a nasal cannula

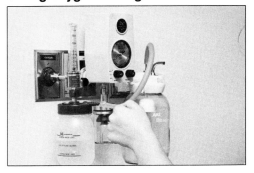

1 *Planning to give your patient humidified oxygen through a nasal cannula? Before you begin, take time to explain the procedure to him. Next, make sure there's enough sterile or distilled water in the humidifier bottle.* Now, as shown in this photo, attach the end of the oxygen tubing to the humidifier's nipple. Set the liter flow to the desired rate. Make sure you can feel oxygen flowing from prongs.

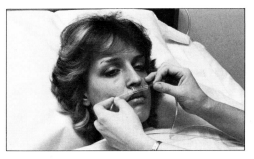

2 Now, place the two prongs of the cannula into the patient's nostrils, as shown, with the tab facing up. Be sure the prongs curve upward.

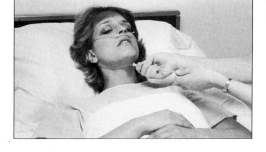

3 Next, position the tubing over and behind each ear. Gently secure it by sliding the adjuster under the chin. Be careful not to adjust the tubing too tightly.

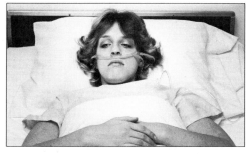

4 Not all cannulas are alike. This type has an elastic strap that fits around the patient's head. If you use this type of cannula, you must adjust the elastic so the cannula's secure, yet comfortable.

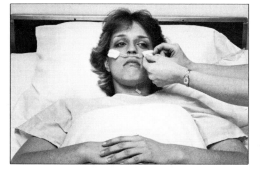

5 The tubing on *any* type of cannula may cause skin irritation. To guard against it, pad the tubing with 2" x 2" gauze pads. Slip the pads under the tubing, as shown, to protect the cheek area. Also slip pads behind the ears or wherever the patient complains of irritation.

How to insert an oxygen catheter

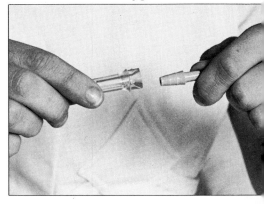

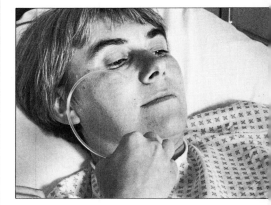

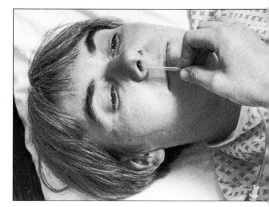

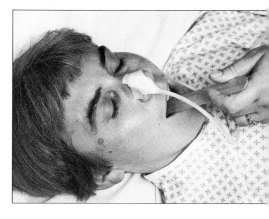

1 *Does your patient need an oxygen catheter inserted in her nose? Here's how to do it:* First, explain what you're going to do. Then, use a penlight to check each nostril for septal deviation or other obstruction. Suction nasal passages, if necessary. Ask the patient to occlude first one nostril, then the other, to see if she can breathe well through each. If both nostrils are obstructed, you'll have to use another method to deliver oxygen.

Now, complete the step shown in this photo. Attach the oxygen catheter to the tube that connects it to the humidified oxygen unit. Make sure the catheter's patent and has no leaks. Keep oxygen flow turned *off* until you've correctly inserted catheter.

2 Next, measure the catheter distance from the patient's earlobe to the tip of her nose. Pinch catheter at that length with your thumb and fingers to mark it.

3 Now, lubricate catheter with sterile water or a water-soluble jelly. Gently insert it into the patient's nostril. If you have difficulty at first, try tilting up the tip of her nose. Continue easing the catheter into the nostril until you've reached the measured distance.

4 Check the catheter's position to make sure it's correct. To do this, hold the patient's tongue down with a tongue blade and examine her throat. If the catheter's correctly positioned, you'll see its tip directly behind the uvula. If you don't see it, chances are you haven't inserted it far enough. Try again.

If that fails, the catheter's probably curled. Pull it out and start over.

Using a simple oxygen mask

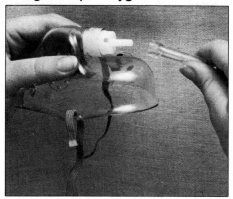

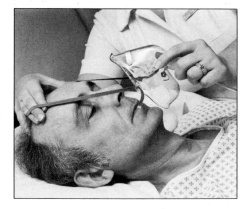

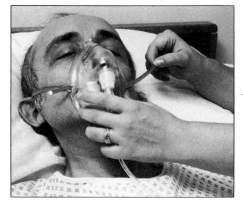

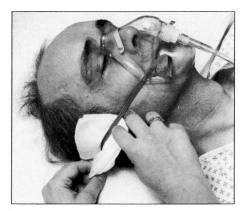

1 *Begin by telling the patient what you're going to do. Explain how the oxygen mask will help him breathe easier, so he won't be frightened by the procedure. When you've answered any questions he has, proceed as follows:* Attach one end of the oxygen supply tube to the mask, as shown, and the other end to the humidifier nipple. Now, turn on the oxygen, beginning with a higher flow than prescribed (about 10 to 15 liters per minute) to momentarily flush the mask. Then, set the flow at the prescribed level.

2 Gently place the mask over the patient's face. Slip the loosened elastic strap over his head so it's positioned either below or above his ears.

3 Pull the ends of the elastic, as shown, until the mask fits snugly. Make sure it's snug enough to prevent too much room air from diluting the oxygen, but don't make it uncomfortably tight. Adjust the mask's metal nosestrap to fit the patient's face so oxygen won't leak into the patient's eyes. Plug any gaps that remain with gauze pads.

4 *Nursing tip:* Don't let the elastic strap irritate the patient's scalp or ears. To prevent irritation, put 4" x 4" gauze pads under the strap, as shown. Wash and dry the patient's face every 2 hours to reduce irritation. Don't use powder, however, because the patient may inhale it.

Oxygen delivery systems

Using a nonrebreathing mask

A nonrebreathing mask will give your patient the highest oxygen concentration possible, short of positive pressure ventilation or intubation with mechanical ventilation. The one-way valve between the mask and the reservoir prevents the patient's exhaled air from entering the bag. To use it, flush the mask and bag with oxygen *before* you apply it. Then, slip the elastic strap around the back of the patient's head and position it above his ears. Adjust liter flow to prescribed rate. Prevent pressure sores by placing 4" x 4" gauze pads where the strap touches his ears. Adjust the metal strap over his nose. Mold it to fit his face snugly, but not uncomfortably. Keep the bag from twisting or kinking and never allow it to totally deflate with inspiration. Increase the oxygen flow rate if necessary.

Note: If your patient requires long-term oxygen therapy, you'll find the nonrebreathing mask impractical and poorly tolerated.

Also, this may be inadequate for patients with erratic respirations because the bag doesn't have a chance to fill with oxygen between inspirations.

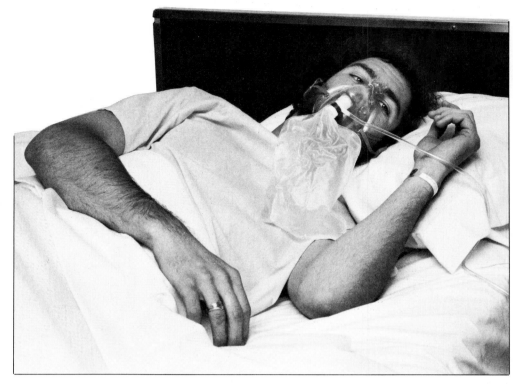

How to convert a nonrebreathing mask into a partial rebreather

A partial rebreathing mask delivers high concentrations of oxygen by allowing your patient to rebreathe the first one third of his exhaled air. Some hospitals stock them, but if your hospital doesn't, you'll have to make one from a nonrebreathing mask. Here's how:

First, remove the rubber flap that's located just inside the mask (over the reservoir bag). Don't remove the rubber flaps on the side portals, because they prevent room air from entering the mask. (They do, however, allow the patient to exhale through them.) *Nursing tip:* Save the rubber flap you did remove in a plastic bag. You may want to replace it later to increase the patient's FIO_2.

To apply the partial rebreather, follow the steps listed for the nonrebreathing mask.

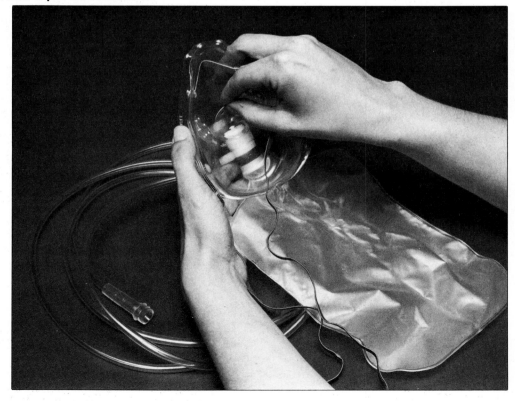

How to assemble a Croupette

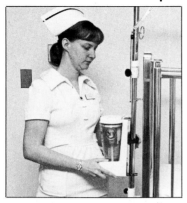

1 *Caring for a small child with a respiratory inflammation like bronchitis? To loosen the child's secretions and help him breathe easier, the doctor may want him placed in a Croupette, which can deliver humidified air or oxygen.* To assemble one kind of Croupette, follow these instructions: First, anchor the Croupette frame to the back of the crib, as shown. Then, attach a nebulizer to it.

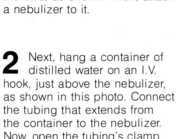

3 Form a tent over the crib by attaching the loops on the plastic canopy to the frame hooks.

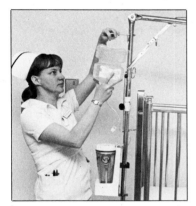

2 Next, hang a container of distilled water on an I.V. hook, just above the nebulizer, as shown in this photo. Connect the tubing that extends from the container to the nebulizer. Now, open the tubing's clamp and fill the nebulizer.

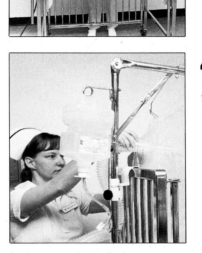

4 When that's completed, place the end of the wide-bore nebulizer tubing into the tent opening provided for it.

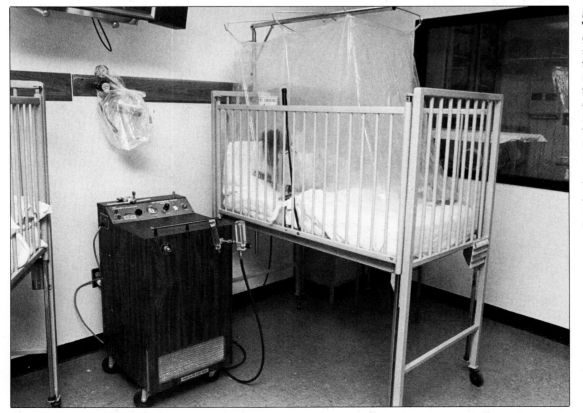

5 Now, connect the Croupette to the unit delivering oxygen or compressed air, as shown here. Tuck the tent under the mattress to prevent humidity loss. When the air inside the tent is heavily misted, place the child inside. Cover him with a bath blanket or large towel to keep him from getting chilled. Replace it immediately if it becomes damp.
Important: Check your patient frequently to make sure the air inside the Croupette is heavily misted. And remember to refill the nebulizer, as needed.

Oxygen delivery systems

Operating an Inspiron venturi mask

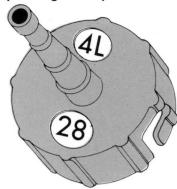

1 *Because the venturi mask delivers a precise concentration of oxygen, it's frequently used on COPD patients. The Inspiron venturi mask is conveniently prepackaged, with wide-bore tubing, jet adapters, and an optional humidification adapter. The jet adapters are color-coded. Each color coincides with a specific liter flow of oxygen and an exact concentration of oxygen.*

Color	Liters per minute	Concentration of oxygen*
Blue	4	24%
Yellow	4	28%
White	6	31%
Green	8	35%
Pink	8	40%
*Some companies have masks using the venturi principle, with jet adapters up to 50%.		

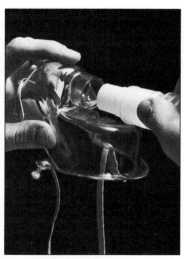

2 Now, here's how to use the venturi mask, which you'll see illustrated in detail on the opposite page. First, attach the male adapter of the mask to the wide-bore tubing.

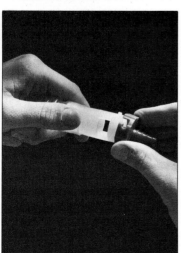

3 Select the prescribed jet adapter, and match the slots to the prongs on the entrainment collector. Push the jet adapter onto the entrainment collector, as shown here. Then, turn the jet adapter clockwise one half turn, locking it in place.

Nursing tip: Always keep the bag of remaining jet adapters at the patient's bedside. The doctor may prescribe a different oxygen concentration because of changes in the patient's blood gas measurements.

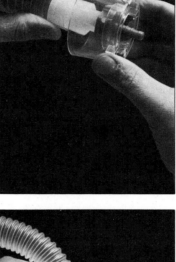

4 Some patients receive only oxygen therapy with the venturi mask. In such cases, attach one end of the oxygen tube to the jet adapter nipple, and twist it in place. Attach the other end of the oxygen tube to the nipple on the oxygen flowmeter.

For patients also requiring humidification, you'll need to attach a humidification adapter to the jet adapter before you attach the oxygen tube. To do this, grasp the wide-bore tubing and slip the humidification adapter over the jet adapter. Keep the chimney straight up. *Remember:* The doctor will usually order humidification if oxygen concentration exceeds 30%.

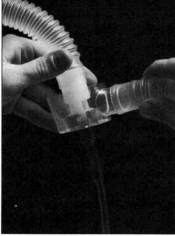

5 Affix one end of the wide-bore tube to the chimney of the humidification adapter, and the other end to the humidifier. Make sure the humidifier contains sterile or distilled water. Next, select the oxygen liter flow by referring to the code on the jet adapter. Flush the tubing with oxygen, and check it for air leaks. Be sure you see an adequate mist coming from humidifier.

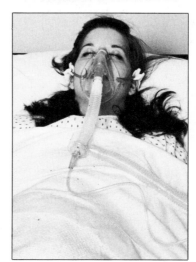

6 Place the venturi mask over the patient's nose and mouth. Slip the elastic strap around the back of the patient's head, and position it above her ears. Prevent pressure sores by placing 4" x 4" gauze pads where the strap touches her ears. Adjust the metal strip over the nose by pinching it into shape. The mask should fit snugly but not uncomfortably. Don't let the wide-bore tubing twist or kink.

For special tips on how to make your patient comfortable, see the opposite page.

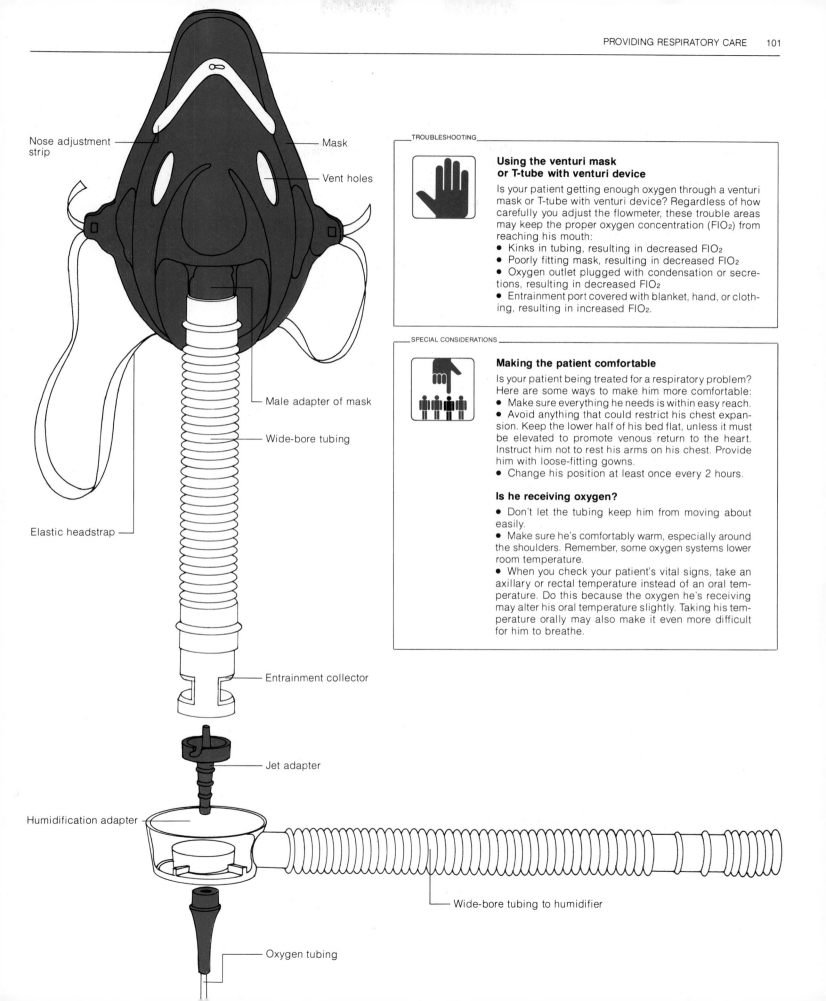

Nose adjustment strip

Mask

Vent holes

Male adapter of mask

Wide-bore tubing

Elastic headstrap

Entrainment collector

Jet adapter

Humidification adapter

Wide-bore tubing to humidifier

Oxygen tubing

**Using the venturi mask
or T-tube with venturi device**

Is your patient getting enough oxygen through a venturi mask or T-tube with venturi device? Regardless of how carefully you adjust the flowmeter, these trouble areas may keep the proper oxygen concentration (FIO_2) from reaching his mouth:
• Kinks in tubing, resulting in decreased FIO_2
• Poorly fitting mask, resulting in decreased FIO_2
• Oxygen outlet plugged with condensation or secretions, resulting in decreased FIO_2
• Entrainment port covered with blanket, hand, or clothing, resulting in increased FIO_2.

Making the patient comfortable

Is your patient being treated for a respiratory problem? Here are some ways to make him more comfortable:
• Make sure everything he needs is within easy reach.
• Avoid anything that could restrict his chest expansion. Keep the lower half of his bed flat, unless it must be elevated to promote venous return to the heart. Instruct him not to rest his arms on his chest. Provide him with loose-fitting gowns.
• Change his position at least once every 2 hours.

Is he receiving oxygen?

• Don't let the tubing keep him from moving about easily.
• Make sure he's comfortably warm, especially around the shoulders. Remember, some oxygen systems lower room temperature.
• When you check your patient's vital signs, take an axillary or rectal temperature instead of an oral temperature. Do this because the oxygen he's receiving may alter his oral temperature slightly. Taking his temperature orally may also make it even more difficult for him to breathe.

Oxygen delivery systems

Attaching a T-piece to a venturi system

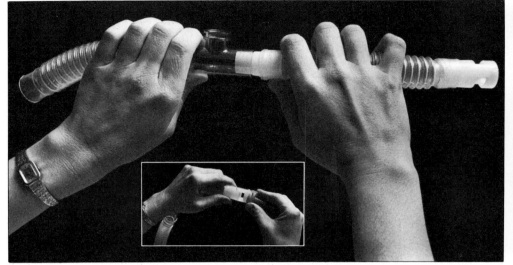

1 *Imagine that you're caring for a patient with a trach or endotracheal tube. If she's being weaned or her breathing becomes so difficult that she requires oxygen, you may have to use a T-piece to hook the tube to a venturi system.*

Here's how: First, attach the short piece of wide-bore tubing that comes with the venturi to one end of a T-tube. Attach a 6" piece of wide-bore tubing to the other end.

[Inset] Now, connect the jet adapter with the prescribed oxygen concentration to the venturi tube's entrainment collector, as shown in this photo. Turn it clockwise to lock it in place.

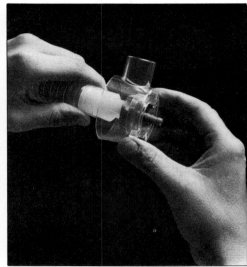

2 Next, attach the humidification adapter to the jet adapter, as the nurse is doing in this photo.

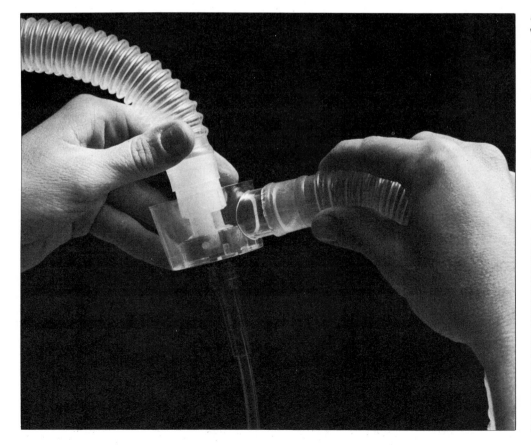

3 Follow that step by attaching an oxygen tube to the jet adapter's nipple. Now, connect a long piece of wide-bore tubing to the humidification adapter, as we show here. Turn oxygen to prescribed flow rate, and adjust humidifier to get adequate mist.

4 When these steps are complete, you can attach the open end of the T-piece to the patient's trach tube, as the nurse has done in this photo. Reassure your patient by explaining why the equipment is necessary and how it will help her breathe more easily.

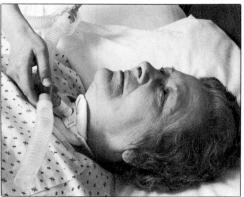

Applying a trach collar

1 To deliver oxygen to a patient with a tracheostomy, you can use a trach collar, or what's sometimes called a trach mask.

Here's how: First, attach the large-bore tubing that comes from the oxygen or compressed air unit to the swivel adapter on the collar. Next, set the oxygen or air to the prescribed flow rate and concentration. Check the tubing's patency. Be sure the oxygen or air is humidified, because you're bypassing the patient's upper airways, which normally humidify it for her.

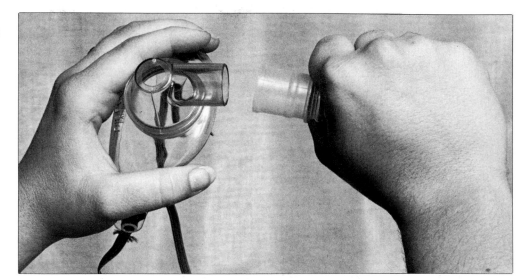

2 Snap the elastic strap on one side of the collar, as shown. Now, place the collar's center opening directly over the patient's trach tube.

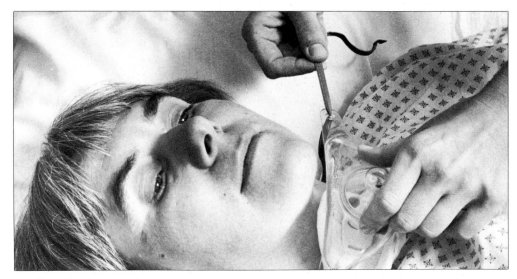

3 Slip the free end of the strap around the back of your patient's neck, and insert it through the opening on the collar's other side. Adjust it by pulling gently.

Now, position the wide-bore tubing, remembering that you can move the swivel adapter to either side. Take care not to block the exhalation port with bed linen.

Nursing tip: Planning to suction a patient who's wearing a trach collar? You don't need to remove it; just suction through the opening in the collar, being careful not to contaminate the catheter. Hyperinflate patient's lungs before and after procedure.

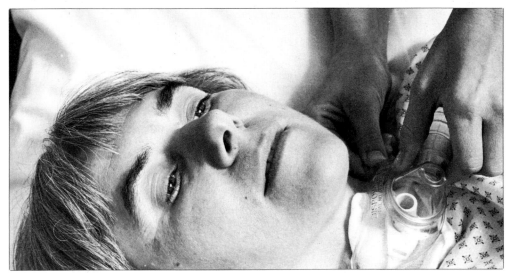

Oxygen delivery systems

What you should know about low- and high-flow oxygen delivery systems

Apparatus	Benefits	Problems to expect	To avoid complications
Nasal cannula (Low-flow system)	• Safe and simple • Comfortable; easily tolerated • Nasal prongs can be shaped to fit facial contour. • Effective for delivering low oxygen concentrations • Allows freedom of movement; doesn't interfere with eating or talking • Inexpensive; disposable • Can provide continuous, positive airway pressure for infants and children.	• Can't deliver oxygen concentrations greater than 40% • Can't be used when patient has complete nasal obstructions; for example, mucosal edema or polyps • May cause headaches or dry mucous membranes if flow rate exceeds 6 liters per minute • Can dislodge easily • Strap may pinch chin if adjusted too tightly. • Patient must be alert and cooperative to help keep cannula in place.	• Remove and clean cannula every 8 hours with a wet cloth. Give good mouth and nose care. • If patient's restless, tape cannula in place. • Check for pressure areas under nose and over ears. Apply gauze padding, if necessary. • Moisten lips and nose with lubricating jelly, but take care not to occlude cannula.
Nasal catheter (Low-flow system)	• Allows freedom of movement; doesn't interfere with eating or talking • Provides stable delivery if patient's restless • Inexpensive; disposable • Doubles as a suction catheter.	• Can't deliver oxygen concentrations greater than 45% • May cause headaches or sinus pain if flow rate exceeds 6 liters per minute • May dry nostrils and mucous membranes • Catheter lumen may clog with secretions. • Kinks easily • Less comfortable than nasal cannula; tape may irritate skin. • Patients lacking epiglottal reflexes may experience abdominal distention, especially at high-flow rates.	• Change catheter every 8 hours, alternating nostrils; give good mouth and nose care. • Check for skin irritation caused by tape. • Use for short-term therapy. • Moisten nose with lubricating jelly. • Use with caution in comatose or debilitated patients.
Simple face mask (Low-flow system)	• Effectively delivers high oxygen concentrations • Humidification can be increased by using large-bore tubing and aerosol mask. • Doesn't dry mucous membranes of nose and mouth.	• Hot and confining; may irritate skin • Tight seal, necessary for higher oxygen concentration, may cause discomfort. • Interferes with eating and talking • Can't deliver less than 40% oxygen • Impractical for long-term therapy.	• Don't use on patient with COPD. • Place pads between mask and boney facial parts. • Periodically massage face with fingertips. • Wash and dry face every 2 hours. • For adequate flush, maintain flow rate of 5 liters per minute. • Don't adjust strap too tightly. • Remove and clean mask every 8 hours with a wet cloth.

What you should know about low- and high-flow oxygen delivery systems continued

Apparatus	Benefits	Problems to expect	To avoid complications
Face tent (High- or low-flow system)	• Provides high humidity • Functions as a high-flow system when attached to a venturi nebulizer • Substitutes for face mask if patient can't tolerate having his nose covered; for example, if his nose is broken • Doesn't dry mucous membranes.	• Hot and confining; may irritate skin • Interferes with eating and talking • Doesn't deliver precise oxygen concentrations without venturi attachment; patient can rebreathe CO_2 unless venturi system is used. • Impractical for long-term therapy.	• Same as for simple face mask • Watch for signs of oxygen toxicity, especially when a venturi attachment is not used.
Partial rebreathing mask (Low-flow system)	• Oxygen reservoir bag lets patient rebreathe his exhaled air, which is high in oxygen content. This increases his fraction inspired oxygen concentration (FIO_2). • Safety valve allows room air to be inhaled if oxygen source fails. • Effectively delivers higher oxygen concentrations (35% to 60%) • Easily humidifies oxygen • Doesn't dry mucous membranes • By inserting a rubber flange over the reservoir bag, you can convert most types to nonrebreather masks.	• Tight seal, necessary to ensure accurate oxygen concentrations, may cause discomfort. • Interferes with eating and talking • Hot and confining; may irritate skin • Bag may twist or kink. • Impractical for long-term therapy.	• Never let bag totally deflate during inhalation. Increase liter flow, if necessary. • Avoid twisting bag. • Keep mask snug to prevent inhalation of room air. • To initially fill bag, apply mask as patient exhales.
Nonrebreathing mask (Low-flow system)	• Delivers the highest possible oxygen concentration (60% to 90%) short of intubation and mechanical ventilation • Effective for short-term therapy • Doesn't dry mucous membranes • Can be converted to a partial rebreathing mask, if necessary.	• Requires a tight seal, which may be difficult to maintain; may cause discomfort • May irritate skin • Impractical for long-term therapy.	• Never let bag totally deflate. • Avoid twisting bag. • Keep mask snug to prevent inhalation of room air. • Make sure that all rubber flaps remain in place. • Watch patient closely for signs of oxygen toxicity.
Trach collar or mask (Low-flow system)	• Provides high humidity • Swivel adapter allows tubing to attach on either side. • Frontal port permits suctioning. • Elastic ties allow you to pull mask from tracheostomy without removing it.	• If condensation's allowed to collect, it can drain into tracheostomy. • If secretions collect in the collar, stoma can become infected. • Heated aerosol may cause bleeding if used on fresh trach. • Intake of room air through the port lowers oxygen concentration.	• Empty condensation buildup at least once every 2 hours. • Remove and clean mask every 4 hours with *water*. • Don't cover exhalation port. • Make sure nebulizer delivers constant mist.

Oxygen delivery systems

What you should know about low- and high-flow oxygen delivery systems continued

Apparatus	Benefits	Problems to expect	To avoid complications
T-tube (Low- or high-flow system)	• Chimney extension functions as partial rebreather. • Offers high humidity • Allows greater patient mobility • Can be used for trach or endotrach • Functions as a high-flow system when attached to a venturi system.	• May stick to tracheostomy (from humidity or secretions) • Condensation can collect in tube and drain into tracheostomy.	• If tube sticks to tracheostomy, gently twist off. Then, clean tube with hydrogen peroxide, rinse with water and replace. • Empty condensation buildup at least once every 2 hours. • Keep chimney extension in place. If you don't, the fraction inspired oxygen concentration (FIO_2) will drop drastically. • Make sure humidifier or nebulizer has enough water to create mist. • Watch for signs of oxygen toxicity, especially if used as a low-flow system.
Oxygen hood (Low- or high-flow system)	• Enclosed and compact • Provides more precise oxygen concentration than isolette can by itself. Lets you care for infant's lower torso while upper torso's inside hood. • Functions as a high-flow system when connected to a venturi delivery system • Offers high humidity.	• Can irritate skin • Must be used with a nebulizer • Can't feed infant while he's inside hood • Active infant can move hood.	• Pad hood with towel or foam rubber. • Keep bedding around head dry. • Empty condensation buildup from tubing every 2 hours. • When using heated nebulizer, check hood temperature every 4 hours so it stays between 94° F. (34.4° C.) and 96° F. (35.6° C.).
Isolette (standard) (Low- or high-flow system)	• Provides controlled temperature and humidity • Isolates infants with contagious diseases • Can be used as a high-flow oxygen system to deliver precise oxygen concentrations through an oxygen hood. (To do this, you insert the oxygen tubing through the sleeve at the end port of the isolette.)	• When used without oxygen hood, isolette can deliver only 40% or 100% oxygen. Also, oxygen concentration can fluctuate.	• If 100% oxygen concentration is desired, keep port flaps closed tightly. • If oxygen hood isn't used, check oxygen concentration every 4 hours. • If you're using an oxygen hood with isolette, see instructions listed above.
Croupette (Low-flow system)	• Usually used for children • Delivers high humidity and aerosolized therapy • Allows child to move freely • Disposable canopy.	• If you must open tent, for any reason, remember it'll take 15 to 20 minutes to restore oxygen concentration. • Water or ice reservoir must be filled every 6 to 8 hours. • High humidity promotes bacterial growth. • Isolates patient.	• Check temperature and oxygen concentration every 4 hours. • Use rubber sheet on bed, under linen, to prevent oxygen from escaping through mattress. • Use bath blanket over bottom sheet to absorb excess moisture; change linen and gown every 2 hours to keep patient warm and dry. • Give patient care through tent opening whenever possible. When giving bath or changing linen, tuck tent under pillow to conserve oxygen. • Prevent patient from feeling isolated by talking to him. Use a normal tone; the tent doesn't impair hearing.

What you should know about low- and high-flow oxygen delivery systems continued

Apparatus	Benefits	Problems to expect	To avoid complications
Oxygen tent (Low-flow system)	• Provides high humidity; temperature can be evenly controlled. • Delivers oxygen to severely burned patients without need for an irritating face mask.	• If you must open tent, for any reason, remember it'll take 15 or 20 minutes to restore oxygen concentration. • High humidity promotes bacterial growth. • Condensation may collect in tubing. Empty it at least once every 4 hours. • Isolates patient.	• Use rubber sheet on bed, under linen, to prevent oxygen from escaping through mattress. • Maintain oxygen flow at 10 to 15 liters per minute for adequate flush. • Check temperature and oxygen concentration every 4 hours; check for leaks in tent. • Keep patient warm and dry. Give patient care through tent opening whenever possible. When giving bath or changing linen, tuck tent under pillow to conserve oxygen. • Prevent patient from feeling isolated by talking to him. Use a normal tone; the tent doesn't impair hearing.
Venturi mask (High-flow system)	• Delivers exact oxygen concentrations despite patient's respiratory pattern • Diluter jets can be changed, or dial turned, to change oxygen concentration. • Doesn't dry mucous membranes • Can be used to deliver humidity or aerosol therapy • Never delivers more than the prescribed oxygen concentration, even if knob on flowmeter is accidentally bumped and liter flow is increased.	• Hot and confining; mask may irritate skin. • Fraction inspired oxygen concentration (FIO_2) may be altered if mask doesn't fit snugly, if tubing's kinked, if oxygen intake ports are blocked, or if less than recommended liter flow is used. • Interferes with eating and talking • Condensation may collect and drain on patient if humidification is being used.	• Check arterial blood gas measurements frequently. • Soften skin around mouth with petroleum jelly to prevent irritation. • Remove and clean mask every 8 hours with a wet cloth.

Determining oxygen percentages by liter flow

Do you want to know the approximate percentage of oxygen (FIO_2) your patient is getting from a low-flow delivery system? Use this chart to tell you. Just line up the *method* you're using to deliver the oxygen with the *number* of liters per minute. *Important:* Keep in mind these figures apply only to patients who are breathing at a normal rate and rhythm.

Method of delivery	Oxygen delivered at 2 liter/min.	Oxygen delivered at 3 liter/min.	Oxygen delivered at 4 liter/min.	Oxygen delivered at 5 liter/min.	Oxygen delivered at 6 liter/min.	Oxygen delivered at 8 liter/min.	Oxygen delivered at 10 liter/min.	Oxygen delivered at 12 liter/min.	Oxygen delivered at 15 liter/min.
Cannula/catheter	23%-28%	28%-30%	32%-36%	40%	max. 44%	X	X	X	X
Simple mask	X	X	X	40%	45%-50%	55%-60%	X	X	X
Partial rebreathing mask	X	X	X	X	35%	45%-50%	60%	60%	60%
Nonrebreathing mask	X	X	X	X	55%-60%	60%-80%	80%-90%	90%	90%
Tent, croupette	X	X	X	X	X	X	30%-40%	40%-50%	50%
Isolette standard use	X	X	X	X	35%-40% (with flag up) 80%-90% (with flag down)	40% (with flag up) 90% (with flag down)	40% (with flag up) 95%-100% (with flag down)	X	X

X—not recommended for use at this liter flow
%—concentration of fraction inspired oxygen concentration (FIO_2)

Patient positioning

Positioning the patient with respiratory problems

Problem	Position like this	Benefits	Nursing tips
Dyspnea		• Allows enhanced thoracic movement • Takes little energy to maintain.	• Encourage foot elevation, if possible, to prevent ankle edema. • Use oxygen tubing long enough to let patient move freely. • *Remember:* When the patient uses the overbed table for support, be sure to lock the wheels.
Abdominal distention or end-of-term pregnancy		• Allows enhanced lung expansion without restricting the abdominal cavity • Takes strain off lower back.	• As an alternate, put patient in supine position, with pillow or rolled towel at small of back.
Unconsciousness		• Allows secretions or vomitus to drain from patient's mouth, decreasing risk of aspiration.	• Keep suction equipment handy. • Turn patient every 2 hours. • Place pad on the pillow to catch secretions. Check for spinal fluid leak by watching for a halo around stains.
Postop thoracotomy with tube		• Permits enhanced chest expansion • Improves chest drainage • Relaxes abdominal muscles by slightly bending knees.	• Be careful not to kink the chest tubes. • Roll pillows behind the patient's back for support. • Never raise a surgical patient's knees. Instead, raise the foot of the bed 20°. • Elevate head of bed 30° to 45° • Keep patient on his operative side as much as possible. If you let him lie on his other side, you may restrict the expansion of his good lung.

Positioning the patient with respiratory problems continued

Problem	Position like this	Benefits	Nursing tips
Postop pneumonectomy		• Keeps fluid from draining into remaining lung, drowning patient.	• Position patient on his operative side by *lifting* him at the shoulders instead of sliding him onto his side. Make sure his dressing stays smooth and flat.
Shock		• Reduces abdominal pressure on diaphragm • Promotes venous return.	• Avoid Trendelenburg position, which increases abdominal pressure on the diaphragm. • Raise the foot of the bed 30°.
Tracheostomy		• Supports patient's neck, and keeps it and trach tube properly aligned.	• Make sure the pillow that inflates the tracheostomy cuff hangs free for easy access. • When your patient's sleeping, check periodically to make sure nothing's blocking his tracheostomy.
Rib fractures		• Splints the area; allows fullest inflation of the uninvolved lung.	• Whenever you use a binder for additional support, be sure to release it every 2 hours so the patient can breathe deeply.

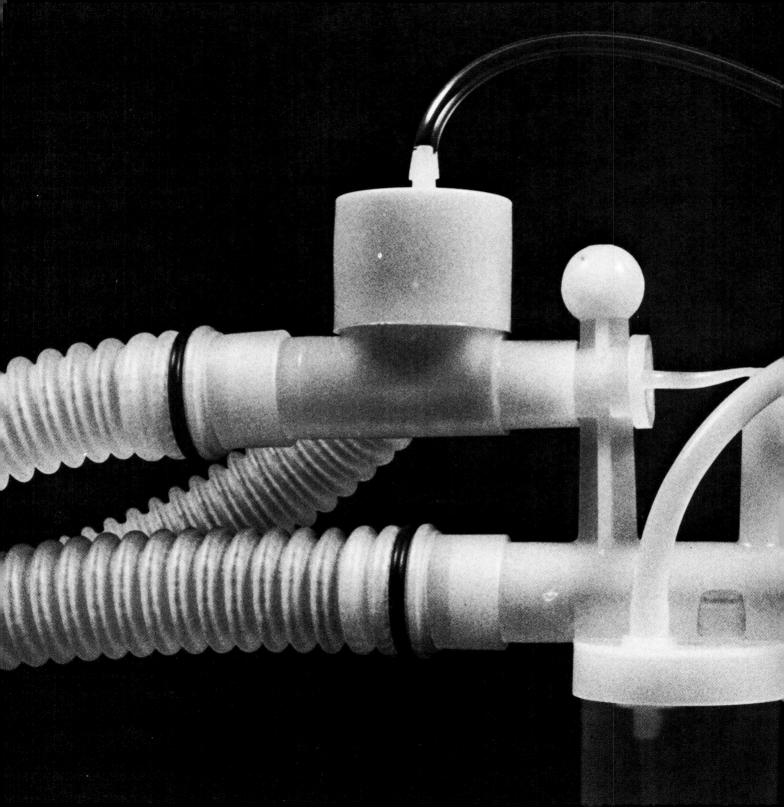

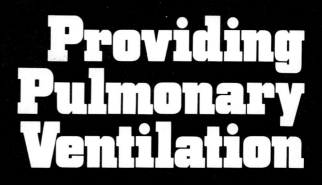

Providing Pulmonary Ventilation

Chest physiotherapy
Postural drainage
Patient teaching
Chest physiotherapy problems
IPPB therapy
Ventilators
Weaning
Special nursing considerations
Phrenic nerve pacer

Chest physiotherapy

You're probably caring for a patient who requires chest physiotherapy. Expect it if he's newly post-op, has cystic fibrosis or COPD, or is receiving mechanical ventilation.

But do you understand how to perform the procedures involved? For example, do you know how to percuss and vibrate the patient's chest adequately? Can you properly position him for postural drainage? Do you know how to teach pursed-lip and diaphragmatic breathing?

If you're not sure, study the information we've included on the following pages. These photostories will show you all the current procedures used in chest physiotherapy and will explain how to avoid some of the problems you'll encounter.

Three different techniques: The whens and hows

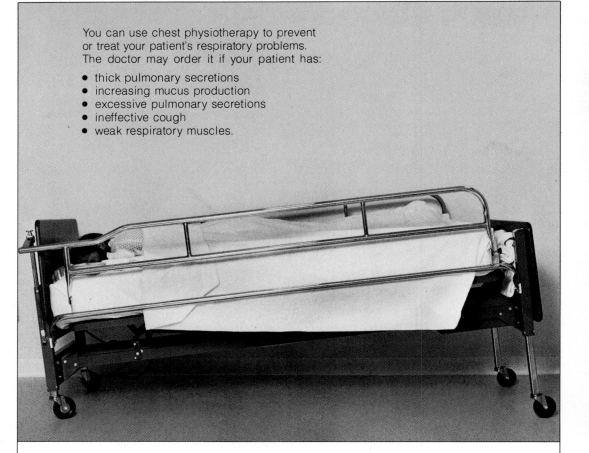

You can use chest physiotherapy to prevent or treat your patient's respiratory problems. The doctor may order it if your patient has:

- thick pulmonary secretions
- increasing mucus production
- excessive pulmonary secretions
- ineffective cough
- weak respiratory muscles.

Technique	Postural drainage
How to perform	Positions for postural drainage vary, depending on which lung segment's involved.
	Place the lung segment to be drained uppermost, with the mainstem bronchus as close to vertical as possible.
Purpose	Enables pulmonary secretions to drain by gravity into the major bronchi or trachea. Then, your patient can dislodge them by coughing. If he can't, he may need percussion and/or vibration techniques.
Nursing considerations	Before you begin, make sure your patient knows how to cough and deep breathe effectively.
	Monitor your patient's cardiac and respiratory status during treatment.
	When you drain lower lobes, decrease the drainage angle if your patient can't tolerate a 30° tilt.
	Don't perform postural drainage immediately after the patient eats.
	Don't use Trendelenburg position if your patient has increased intracranial pressure or acute heart disease.

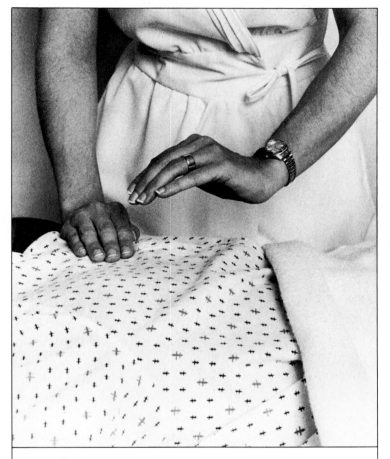

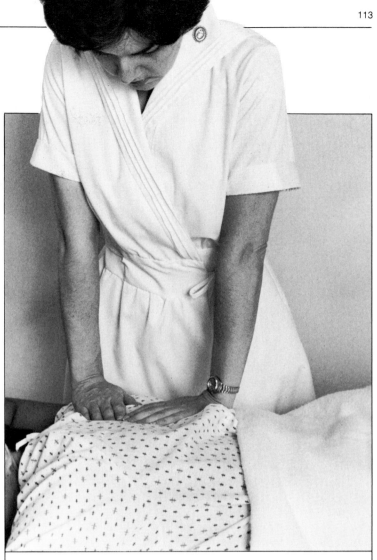

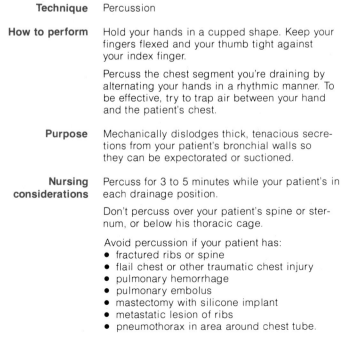

Technique	Percussion
How to perform	Hold your hands in a cupped shape. Keep your fingers flexed and your thumb tight against your index finger.
	Percuss the chest segment you're draining by alternating your hands in a rhythmic manner. To be effective, try to trap air between your hand and the patient's chest.
Purpose	Mechanically dislodges thick, tenacious secretions from your patient's bronchial walls so they can be expectorated or suctioned.
Nursing considerations	Percuss for 3 to 5 minutes while your patient's in each drainage position.
	Don't percuss over your patient's spine or sternum, or below his thoracic cage.
	Avoid percussion if your patient has: • fractured ribs or spine • flail chest or other traumatic chest injury • pulmonary hemorrhage • pulmonary embolus • mastectomy with silicone implant • metastatic lesion of ribs • pneumothorax in area around chest tube.

Technique	Vibration
How to perform	Place your hands flat (side by side with your fingers extended) on the chest segment you're draining.
	Instruct your patient to inhale deeply. Then, as he *slowly exhales,* vibrate his chest by quickly contracting and relaxing the muscles of your arms and shoulders. Stop vibrating when he inhales again. Repeat procedure several times.
Purpose	Increases velocity and turbulence of exhaled air. This loosens secretions and helps propel them into the larger bronchi so they can be expectorated or suctioned.
Nursing considerations	Vibrate your patient's chest in each postural drainage position. If the doctor orders, alternate this method with percussion.
	Use vibration instead of percussion if your patient has extreme pain in chest area, is frail, or has just had thoracic surgery or chest trauma.
	Don't vibrate over your patient's spine or sternum, or below his thoracic cage.
	Try to synchronize vibrations with patient's exhalations.

Postural drainage

How to percuss and drain an adult's lungs

If your patient has pulmonary congestion, the doctor may order postural drainage. Depending on which lung area's involved, you may have to place him in a few, or all, of the following postural drainage positions. If he has thick secretions, the doctor may also order chest percussion. These photos will also show you where to place your hands for proper percussion.

1 Here's how to drain the apical segments of both upper lobes. Have your patient sit on the edge of the bed, with his feet supported. Ask him to tip his head forward slightly. Standing behind him, percuss his upper back and shoulders as close as possible to the apex of his shoulder blades.

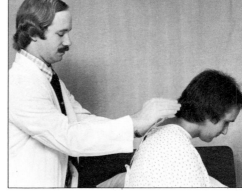

2 To drain the posterior segment of his left upper lobe, raise the head of the bed slightly. Position your patient so he's lying partly on his right side and partly on his abdomen, hugging a pillow, as shown here. Use both hands to percuss the patient's back, near his left scapula. Don't percuss over the boney shoulder blade.

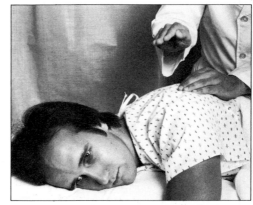

3 To drain the posterior segment of the right upper lobe, lower the bed until it's flat. Position your patient so he's lying partly on his left side and partly on his abdomen, hugging a pillow. Then, percuss his back near his right scapula, as shown here.

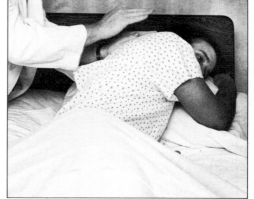

4 To drain the anterior portions of both upper lobes, keep the bed flat. Position your patient on his back. Then, percuss both sides of his upper chest below the clavicle.

When you percuss a woman, work *around* her breasts, not *over* them, to avoid causing pain. If her breasts are too large to percuss around, you may have to use an alternate method to relieve her congestion; for example, postural drainage by itself or postural drainage with mechanical percussor. (For tips on how to use a mechanical percussor, see page 120.)

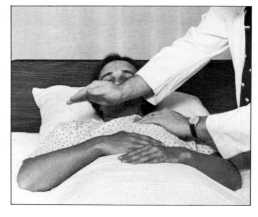

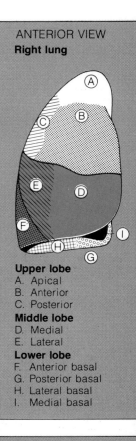

ANTERIOR VIEW
Right lung

Upper lobe
A. Apical
B. Anterior
C. Posterior
Middle lobe
D. Medial
E. Lateral
Lower lobe
F. Anterior basal
G. Posterior basal
H. Lateral basal
I. Medial basal

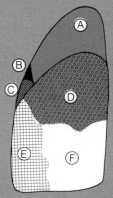

POSTERIOR VIEW
Left lung

Upper lobe
A. Apical posterior
B. Anterior
C. Superior
Lower lobe
D. Superior
E. Lateral basal
F. Posterior basal

Left lung

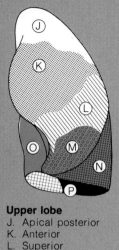

Upper lobe
J. Apical posterior
K. Anterior
L. Superior
M. Inferior
Lower lobe
N. Anteromedial basal
O. Posterior basal
P. Lateral basal

Right lung

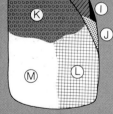

Upper lobe
G. Apical
H. Posterior
I. Anterior
Middle lobe
J. Lateral
Lower lobe
K. Superior
L. Lateral basal
M. Posterior basal

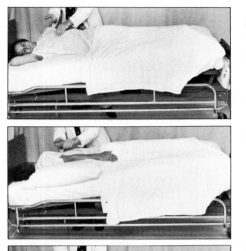

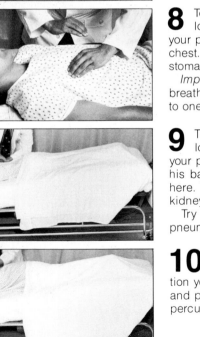

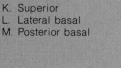

5 To drain the superior and inferior segments of the lingula, elevate the foot of the bed 15°. Position your patient so he's lying partly on his back and partly on his right side. Place a pillow under his left side for support. Then, percuss the left side of his chest between the fourth and sixth ribs. To locate these, feel just above and below the nipple line.

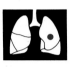

6 To drain the middle lobe of the right lung, raise the foot of the bed 15°. Then, position your patient so he's lying partly on his back and partly on his left side, as shown here. Place a pillow under his back for support. Now, percuss the right side of his chest between the fourth and sixth ribs.

7 To drain the superior segments of both lower lobes, keep the bed flat. Position your patient on his abdomen. Then, as shown here, percuss both sides of his back over the lower ends of his scapulae.

8 To drain the anterior basal segments of both lower lobes, elevate the foot of the bed 30°. Position your patient on his back, and percuss both sides of his chest. *Don't* percuss the center of his chest, over his stomach, because it could cause pain.
Important: An acutely ill patient may have trouble breathing in this position. If he does, adjust bed angle to one he can tolerate. Then, begin percussing.

9 To drain the posterior basal segments of both lower lobes, raise the foot of the bed 30°. Then, position your patient on his abdomen. Percuss both sides of his back at the tenth-rib level and above, as shown here. To avoid causing pain, *don't* percuss over his kidneys, which are located below the tenth-rib level.
Try this position to drain the lungs of a patient with pneumonia.

10 To drain the lateral basal segment of the left lower lobe, elevate the foot of the bed 30°. Position your patient so he's lying partly on his abdomen and partly on his right side, as shown here. Then, percuss his left side at the tenth-rib level and above.

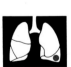

11 To drain the lateral basal segment of the right lower lobe, raise the foot of the bed 30°. Position your patient so he's lying partly on his abdomen and partly on his left side. Then, percuss his right side, as shown here, at the tenth-rib level and above.

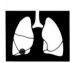

Postural drainage

How to percuss
and drain a toddler's lungs

1 *Begin by observing these guidelines. Hold the child on your lap throughout the procedure to make him more comfortable. Use a pillow for some of the positions. Cover his chest with a T-shirt or pajama top to protect his skin and prevent chilling. To percuss, use three fingers tented together, a small plastic medicine cup, or a padded stethoscope head. Never percuss a child as vigorously as you would an adult.*

Nursing tip: To make the procedure more fun for the child, position him in a colorful beanbag chair and pretend it's a boat.

Here's how to drain the apical segments of the child's upper lung lobes. First, place him in your lap, as shown, and lean him back about 30°. Percuss the area between his collarbone and shoulder blade. Remember to do both sides of his chest.

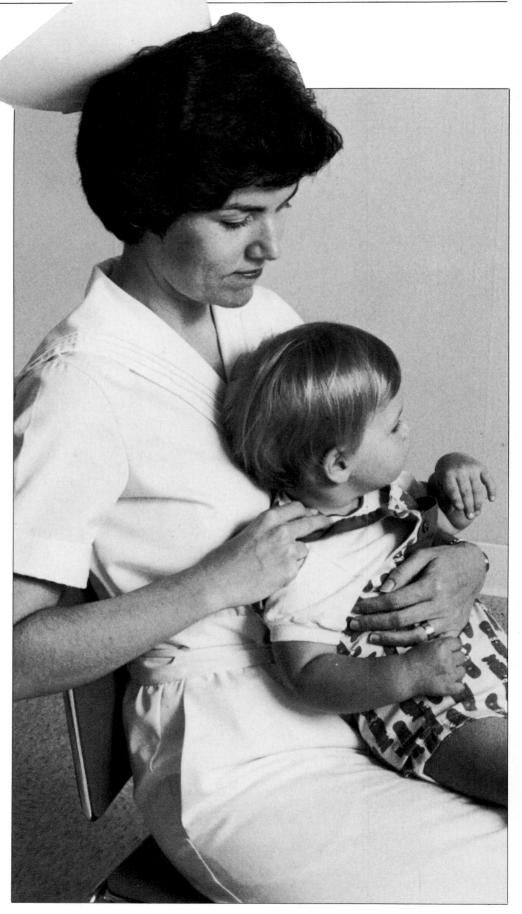

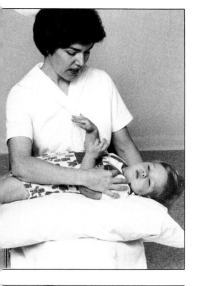

2 Now, put a pillow under the child for the rest of the procedure. To drain the anterior segments of his upper lung lobes, position him on his back, as shown. Percuss between his collarbone and the nipple on each side of his chest.

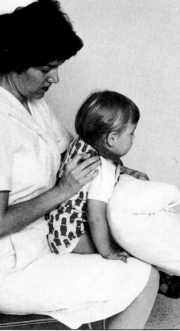

3 To drain the posterior segments of his upper lung lobes, lean the child forward over the pillow. Percuss his upper back on each side.

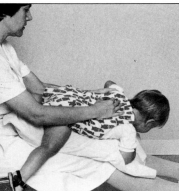

4 To drain the right middle lobe, place the child on his left side with his head lowered about 15°. Now, tip his body slightly backward. Percuss over his right nipple.
   To drain the lingular segment of the left upper lobe, use the same procedure, but place the child on his right side and percuss over his left nipple.

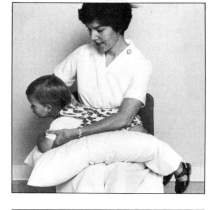

5 To drain the superior segments of his lower lung lobes, place the child flat on his abdomen. Percuss over the middle of his back (below the shoulder blades) on both sides of the spine.

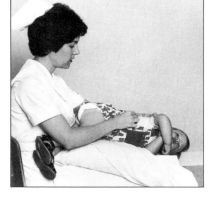

6 To drain the anterior basal segment of the right lower lobe, place the child on his left side, with his head lowered about 30°. Percuss over his right ribs, just beneath his axilla.
   To drain the left anterior basal segment, follow the same procedure, but place the child on his right side. Percuss over his left lower ribs.

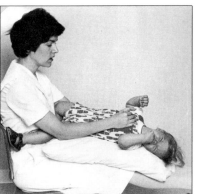

7 To drain the lateral basal segment of the right lower lobe, place the child on his back, with his head lowered about 30°. Now, shift the position of the pillow so his right side is slightly higher than his left. Percuss over the top portion of his right lower ribs.
   To drain the left lateral basal segment, follow the same procedure, but position the child so his left side is higher than his right. Then, percuss over his left lower ribs.

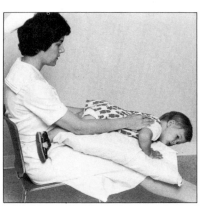

8 To drain the posterior basal segments of the lower lung lobes, place the child flat on his abdomen. Lower his head about 30°. Percuss over his lower ribs, close to his spine. Remember to do both sides.

Patient teaching

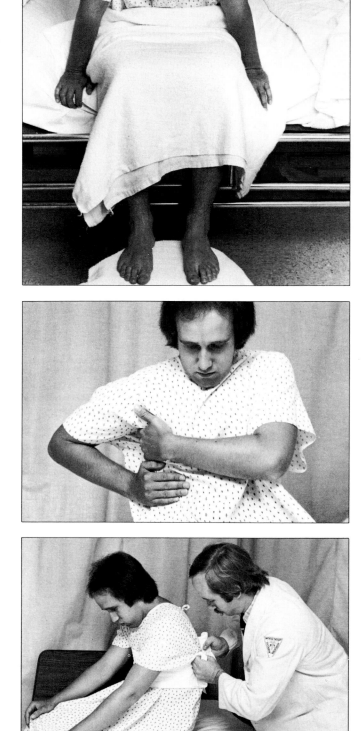

PATIENT TEACHING

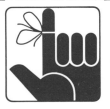

Teaching your patient coughing and splinting

1 *Effective coughing usually helps a patient dislodge pulmonary secretions. To teach your patient how, follow these guidelines:* First, seat him in a chair, or on the edge of his bed, as shown in this photo. Support his feet with a stool if they don't reach the floor. Then, have him hunch his body slightly forward, and tell him to take several slow, deep breaths. Then, instruct your patient to bend his head forward and cough two to three times in rapid succession. Urge him to breathe deeply again, and repeat the entire exercise several times.

2 A patient who's just had surgery should splint his incision before he coughs. Include instructions for splinting in your preop teaching. Show him how to place one hand above and one below his incision, as the patient in this photo is doing. Explain why splinting is important so he'll remember to do it.

3 Suppose your patient has such severe pain after surgery that he can't splint his own incision effectively. Help him. Hold a drawsheet or towel against his incision, as the therapist is doing in this picture. Then, encourage him to deep breathe and cough, as explained.

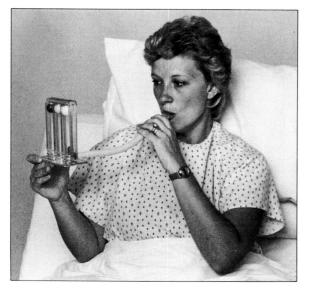

Teaching your patient how to use an incentive spirometer

Suppose a patient who's newly postop finds it difficult or painful to deep breathe. How can you prevent pulmonary complications like atelectasis or pneumonia? Teach him to use an incentive spirometer like the one we've shown here. It may help him put forth more effort. It'll also help both of you determine how effectively he's deep breathing.

How does it work? The flow of air the patient inhales through the mouthpiece of the incentive spirometer is measured by the balls rising in the clear chambers. The TRIFLO® incentive spirometer we show here measures up to 1200 ml of air flow. It has three separate chambers, each measuring a different amount of air.

Here's how to instruct your patient to use the incentive spirometer: First, place him in a seated position, and tell him to hold the incentive spirometer upright. Ask him to exhale normally. Then, tell him to place his lips tightly *around* the mouthpiece and inhale deeply. Unless the doctor's ordered otherwise, encourage the patient to inhale deeply enough to force the ball to the chamber top. Now, instruct him to hold his breath for several seconds, even though the ball will drop. Finally, have him remove the mouthpiece and exhale normally. Repeat the exercise several times, with rests in between. *Remember:* A deep breath held for a few seconds prevents pulmonary complications more effectively than multiple deep breaths that are immediately exhaled.

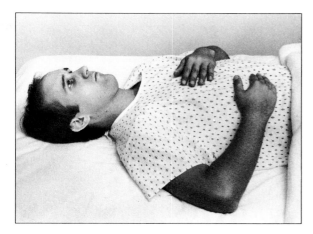

Teaching your patient diaphragmatic breathing

When your patient breathes, are his upper chest muscles doing all the work? If so, teach him to use his diaphragm, as explained below. This technique will increase his breathing capacity, improve ventilation to the lung bases, and decrease his energy expenditure.

Dear Patient:
How to breathe with your diaphragm
Your chest muscles weren't designed to do all the work involved in breathing. You can breathe more efficiently and with less effort if you use your diaphragm and other abdominal muscles. Regular practice is required to train your diaphragm to carry the work load of breathing. At first, you may tire easily. But as you progress, you'll find diaphragmatic breathing's less exhausting than breathing with your chest muscles. Soon, you'll use this technique automatically.

Before beginning the breathing exercise, make sure your nasal passages are clear. If you're congested, blow your nose, and use any medicated aerosol treatment your doctor may have prescribed.

Lie flat on your back, and flex your knees and hips slightly. Now, place one hand over your chest and the other over your upper abdomen. Relax.

With your mouth closed, inhale deeply through your nose. As you do, make your abdomen rise as far as it'll go. Try not to actively expand your chest. If the hand on your abdomen rises as you inhale, you're doing it correctly. Remember, this breathing exercise may take time to master, so don't become discouraged.

Purse your lips, as if you're going to whistle. Exhale *slowly*. While you're exhaling, you may press your lower hand upward to force air from your lungs. Continue this breathing exercise for 10 to 30 minutes, depending on your strength. Stop when you get tired. Repeat the entire exercise at least three to four times daily. Remember to exhale through pursed lips, taking twice as long as you do to inhale.

As soon as you've mastered diaphragmatic breathing while lying flat, try the exercises while standing, and finally while walking. Make it a habit.

Patient teaching

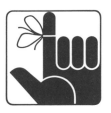

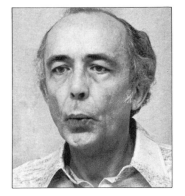

Explaining pursed-lip breathing

Pursed-lip breathing helps patients with COPD empty their alveoli. How? It maintains positive pressure in the airways, keeping them open longer. This enables the patient to exhale more air, which in turn allows him to inhale more air. To teach your patient this breathing technique, place him in a sitting position. Tell him to inhale deeply through his nose. Then, instruct him to exhale with his lips pursed, as shown here.

Remember: To make this technique effective, the patient must exhale *slowly and in a relaxed manner.* If he exhales forcefully, his small airways will probably collapse, trapping more air in the alveoli.

Nursing tip: You'll get better cooperation from a patient if you make a game of it. To do this, fill a glass one-third full with colored water. Give your patient a straw, and let him blow bubbles for 3 minutes, three to four times daily. Make sure he uses his abdominal muscles during exhalation, not his cheeks.

Using a mechanical percussor

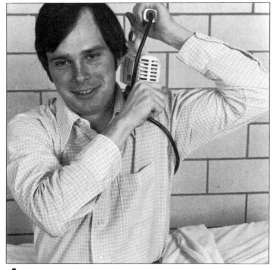

1 *Are you caring for a COPD patient who's about to be discharged from the hospital? The doctor may want him to learn how to percuss himself at home with a mechanical percussor.*

Teach the patient how to use one. Explain what the percussor does and how it can help him. Have the patient try it. In this photo, we show how to percuss over the apical segment of a left upper lobe.

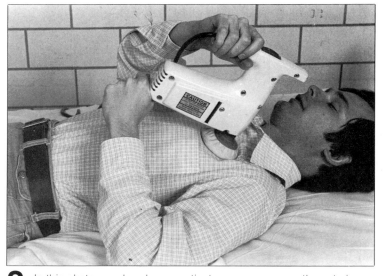

2 In this photo, we show how a patient can percuss over the anterior segment of his left upper lobe. Notice how firmly he grasps the percussor. Tell your patient he'll have better control over it if he holds it with both hands.

Keep in mind that a mechanical percussor weighs about 5 lbs. (2.25 Kg). A frail or weak patient may need someone to help him.

Important: Warn your patient not to use his percussor while he's receiving high concentrations of oxygen. The percussor motor may throw off sparks, which could cause an explosion.

Chest physiotherapy problems

Coping with common problems

Problem
Your patient, who's newly postop, won't practice deep breathing because it's too painful.

Here's what to do
• Reinforce your preop teaching. Explain why deep breathing is necessary to prevent pulmonary complications.
• Make sure he's positioned correctly: Instruct him to sit with his body hunched forward and his neck bent.
• Splint his operative site with a pillow, drawsheet, or show him where to place his hands.
• Force him to take an automatic deep breath by having him exhale completely.

To avoid the problem next time
• Give him the ordered analgesic before you start deep-breathing exercises.
• Encourage him to use an incentive spirometer like the one pictured on page 119.

Problem
You know how to vibrate a chest correctly, but you're not sure how to do it when the patient's on a ventilator.

Here's what to do
• Vibrate only during the ventilator's expiratory phase. During vibration, use the ventilator's sighing mechanism to ensure deep breaths. If the ventilator doesn't have a sighing mechanism, hyperventilate the patient's lungs with a hand-held resuscitator.

To avoid the problem next time
• Review your technique. Make sure you incorporate the above changes.

Problem
Because your patient has signs of lung consolidation, you suspect he isn't coughing effectively.

Here's what to do
• Check the progress notes. Has his cough been productive? *Nursing tip:* Give him a sputum cup to cough into instead of tissues. Note and record the exact amount and color of secretions for comparison with later results.
• If he's postop, make sure he's splinting his operative site correctly.
• Check his position. Is he leaning forward when he coughs?
• Place your hands over his abdomen. Make sure it contracts when he coughs. To assist, press upward and inward on his abdomen.
• Urge him to take several deep breaths to produce a cough.
• Encourage him to cough several times as he exhales.
• If, after these measures, he still doesn't cough effectively, percuss and vibrate him manually.

To avoid the problem next time
• Make sure he gets the necessary patient teaching about proper coughing.
• Give him the ordered analgesic to reduce pain. However, remember that codeine will suppress his cough reflex.

Problem
Your patient complains of pain when you percuss one of his chest areas.

Here's what to do
Make sure you're percussing his chest correctly (see guidelines below).
• Check his skin for redness in the area you're percussing. You may be irritating his skin (see guidelines below).
• If patient's skin isn't red, assess his pain. Does he complain of tenderness when you press on it? Do you feel a lesion or mass beneath his skin? Does his pain increase with inspiration? With coughing? Is he short of breath?
• Document your findings on the patient's chart. Specify the exact location of pain. Observe him closely each time you percuss. Chart any changes in pain or in tolerance to the procedure.
• If he's short of breath, notify the doctor immediately.

To avoid the problem next time
• Examine your technique. (A popping, hollow sound indicates you've created the necessary air cushion.) Make sure you're percussing, not slapping. Keep your fingers flexed and your hands cupped. Relax your upper arms, with most movement coming from your wrists.
• Cover his chest with a towel before percussion, to prevent skin irritation.

IPPB therapy

If you work in a regular medical/ surgical unit, you probably don't see many patients on ventilators. And when you do, you're uncertain how to care for them. You don't understand how basic ventilators differ, or what to do when they malfunction.

This section will help you. In it, we'll:
• introduce the most common ventilators and explain how they work.
• show you how to cope with problems that may develop.
• teach you how to assess when your patient's ready for weaning from the ventilator.
• explain how to help your patient through the weaning process.

INDICATIONS/CONTRAINDICATIONS

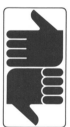

Intermittent positive-pressure breathing (IPPB) therapy

The doctor may want your patient to have IPPB therapy to:
• prevent or treat atelectasis
• augment bronchodilation
• loosen secretions
• deliver deep aerosol therapy
• ease his breathing by reducing PaCO₂ (in some COPD patients)
• treat pulmonary edema.

The doctor probably won't order IPPB therapy if your patient has:
• acute pneumothorax
• subcutaneous or mediastinal emphysema
• tracheoesophageal fistula
• bullous lung disease
• cardiovascular insufficiency (hypotension, hypovolemia, or arrhythmias).

The doctor may also avoid IPPB treatments if the patient won't use the equipment correctly, if treatments cause him distress, or if a less complicated therapy will work.

Setting up an IPPB ventilator

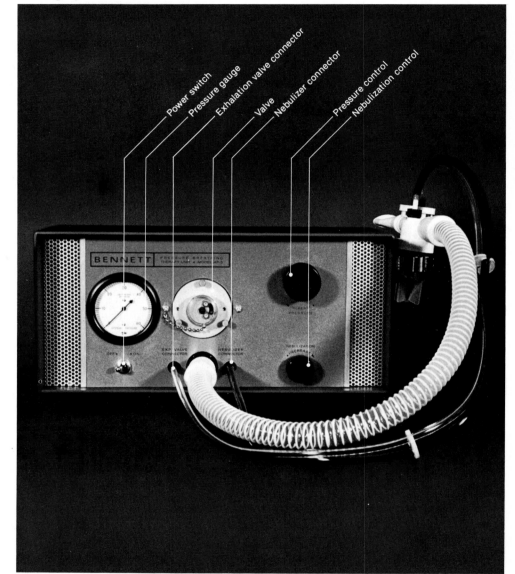

Power switch — Pressure gauge — Exhalation valve connector — Valve — Nebulizer connector — Pressure control — Nebulization control

Giving IPPB treatments to your patient? You may find yourself using a different machine than those pictured on these two pages. However, the principles of operation and patient considerations remain the same. Before administering such therapy, review the indications and contraindications for IPPB treatments listed to the left. You may also want to read about the drugs used for humidification and nebulization therapy on page 94.

1 Here's the Puritan-Bennett AP5. This machine's used only for IPPB treatments, but it can operate on oxygen or room air. (If oxygen is ordered, add it by attaching the nebulizer hose to an oxygen source.) To give IPPB treatments with either room air or oxygen, follow these steps:

• First, attach the tubing as shown here. Then, remove the nebulizer cup, and fill it with the prescribed medicine. *Remember:* Use distilled water to provide humidity if medication isn't ordered.
• Make sure the machine's plugged in. Turn on the power switch. Then, open the nebulizer control knob until you see a light mist coming from the mouthpiece.
• Now, turn the pressure control knob clockwise to a low setting (less than 10). As the patient inhales through the mouthpiece, adjust the knob so the pressure gauge records the prescribed pressure at the end of inspiration.
• Begin the IPPB treatment as explained in the patient teaching aid on the opposite page.

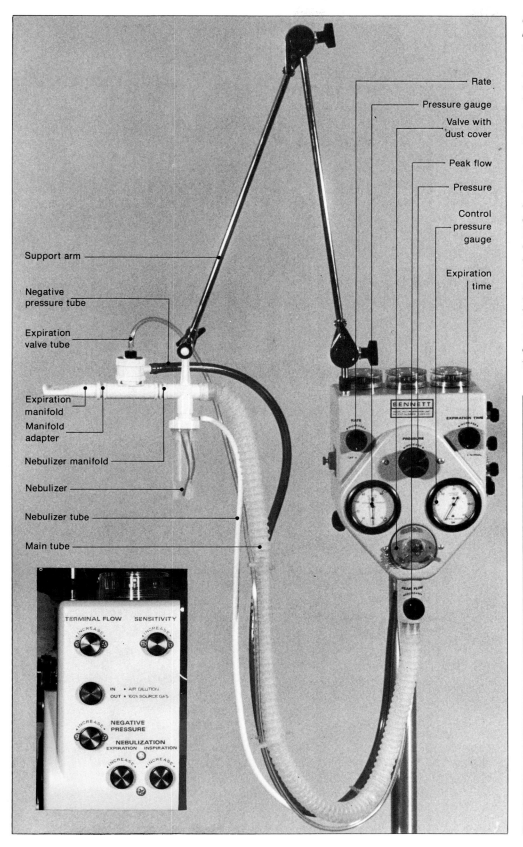

Support arm

Negative
pressure tube

Expiration
valve tube

Expiration
manifold

Manifold
adapter

Nebulizer manifold

Nebulizer

Nebulizer tube

Main tube

Rate

Pressure gauge

Valve with
dust cover

Peak flow

Pressure

Control
pressure
gauge

Expiration
time

2 The Puritan-Bennett PR2, shown here, delivers either IPPB treatments or controlled ventilation to the patient. Here's how to prepare the machine for IPPB therapy:
• First, make sure the ventilation rate is turned off. The patient controls the rate during IPPB.
• After attaching the tubing, as shown here, unscrew the nebulizer cup. Place the prescribed medication inside the cup and replace it tightly. *Remember:* Never give a dry treatment; use distilled water to provide humidity if medication isn't ordered.
• Next, connect the pressure hose to the oxygen wall outlet. Turn the pressure control knob clockwise until the gauge reads the ordered pressure. To avoid delivering 100% oxygen, push the oxygen concentration knob all the way in. You'll now get a mixture of air and oxygen.
• Remove the dust cap from the valve. Lift the drum pin, and adjust the inspiration nebulization button until you see a light mist in the nebulizer cup.
• Begin the IPPB treatment as explained in the patient teaching aid below.

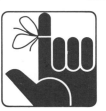

Ventilators

Understanding mechanical ventilator cycles

When a patient needs help breathing, he may be put on a mechanical ventilator which will simulate the normal bellows action usually provided by his diaphragm and thoracic cage.

What type of ventilator the doctor will choose depends on the patient's specific needs. Ventilators are classified by function, based on the variables they deliver during certain phases of the cycle shown in the illustration below. Study it carefully. It'll help you identify ventilator cycles and correspond them with the information on the opposite page.

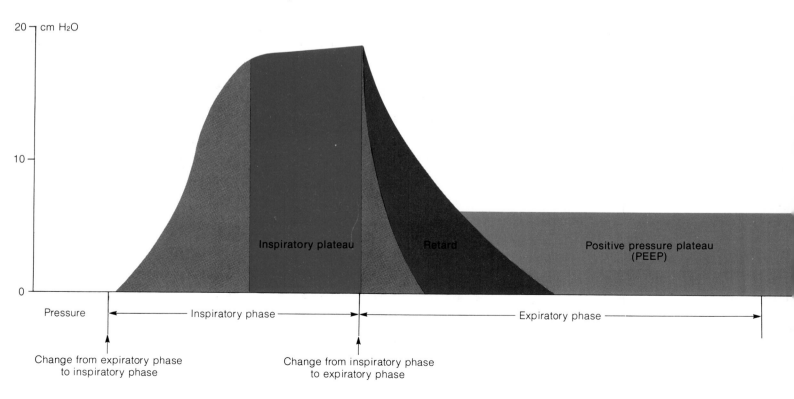

PHASES OF THE MECHANICAL VENTILATOR CYCLE WITH AND WITHOUT PEEP AND RETARD

Getting acquainted with the MA-1 ventilator

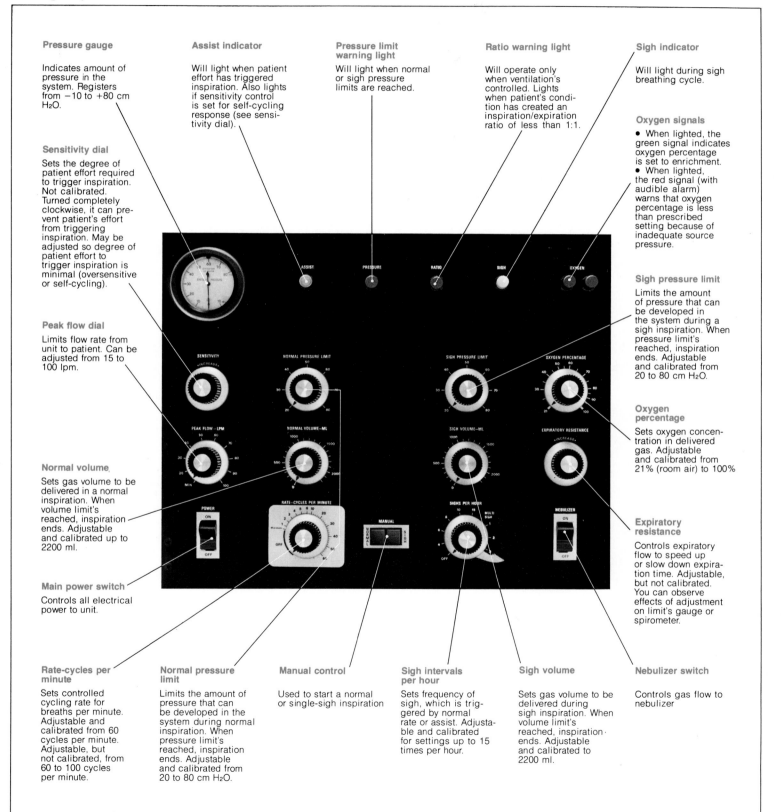

Pressure gauge

Indicates amount of pressure in the system. Registers from −10 to +80 cm H_2O.

Sensitivity dial

Sets the degree of patient effort required to trigger inspiration. Not calibrated. Turned completely clockwise, it can prevent patient's effort from triggering inspiration. May be adjusted so degree of patient effort to trigger inspiration is minimal (oversensitive or self-cycling).

Peak flow dial

Limits flow rate from unit to patient. Can be adjusted from 15 to 100 lpm.

Normal volume

Sets gas volume to be delivered in a normal inspiration. When volume limit's reached, inspiration ends. Adjustable and calibrated up to 2200 ml.

Main power switch

Controls all electrical power to unit.

Assist indicator

Will light when patient effort has triggered inspiration. Also lights if sensitivity control is set for self-cycling response (see sensitivity dial).

Pressure limit warning light

Will light when normal or sigh pressure limits are reached.

Ratio warning light

Will operate only when ventilation's controlled. Lights when patient's condition has created an inspiration/expiration ratio of less than 1:1.

Sigh indicator

Will light during sigh breathing cycle.

Oxygen signals

• When lighted, the green signal indicates oxygen percentage is set to enrichment.
• When lighted, the red signal (with audible alarm) warns that oxygen percentage is less than prescribed setting because of inadequate source pressure.

Sigh pressure limit

Limits the amount of pressure that can be developed in the system during a sigh inspiration. When pressure limit's reached, inspiration ends. Adjustable and calibrated from 20 to 80 cm H_2O.

Oxygen percentage

Sets oxygen concentration in delivered gas. Adjustable and calibrated from 21% (room air) to 100%

Expiratory resistance

Controls expiratory flow to speed up or slow down expiration time. Adjustable, but not calibrated. You can observe effects of adjustment on limit's gauge or spirometer.

Rate-cycles per minute

Sets controlled cycling rate for breaths per minute. Adjustable and calibrated from 60 cycles per minute. Adjustable, but not calibrated, from 60 to 100 cycles per minute.

Normal pressure limit

Limits the amount of pressure that can be developed in the system during normal inspiration. When pressure limit's reached, inspiration ends. Adjustable and calibrated from 20 to 80 cm H_2O.

Manual control

Used to start a normal or single-sigh inspiration

Sigh intervals per hour

Sets frequency of sigh, which is triggered by normal rate or assist. Adjustable and calibrated for settings up to 15 times per hour.

Sigh volume

Sets gas volume to be delivered during sigh inspiration. When volume limit's reached, inspiration ends. Adjustable and calibrated to 2200 ml.

Nebulizer switch

Controls gas flow to nebulizer

Ventilators

How to set up an MA-1 ventilator

1 *The time is 3:00 a.m. Your patient needs a ventilator and no respiratory technician's available. What do you do? Can you set up the ventilator properly by yourself? This photostory will show you how.*

In the photo below you'll see the Puritan-Bennett MA-I ventilator with tubes unattached. To make it functional, you'll need a *ventilator tube kit* from central supply. Check to see that it contains everything you need to make the ventilator work: wide-bore tubing (with appropriate attachments), connectors, and a manifold/nebulizer unit.

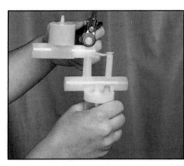

2 Now, fill the cascade humidifier bowl with sterile water to the level marked "full." *Don't* use a saline solution; the salt will damage the machine. Screw the water reservoir tightly to the lid, as shown in the photo.

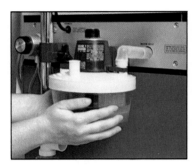

3 Next, look for the ball on top of the manifold/nebulizer unit, and connect it to the ventilator's support arm.

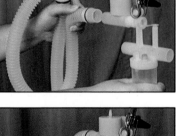

4 Pick up the wide-bore tube that's joined by a Y-connector. Attach one port just below the exhalation valve, as the nurse is doing in the photo.

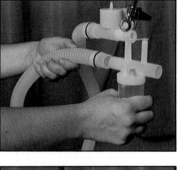

5 Attach the Y-tube's other end to the manifold's inspiratory port, near the nebulizer cup.

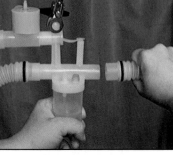

6 Now, pick up the wide-bore tube that has two thin tubes attached to it: clear and white. Connect one end of the wide-bore tube to the nebulizer cup's inspiratory port, as shown in this photo.

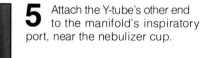

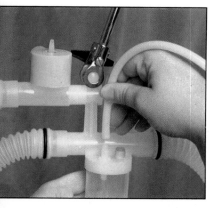

7 Attach the white tube to the nebulizer cup, as shown in this photo.

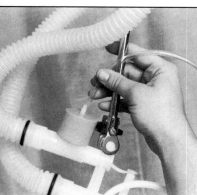

8 Then, attach the clear tube to the exhalation valve nipple.

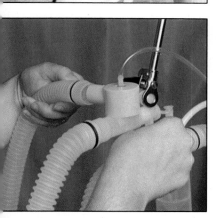

9 Next, take the remaining section of wide-bore tubing and attach one end of it to the exhalation valve port.

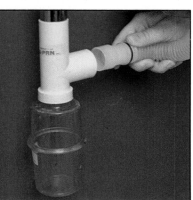

10 Attach the wide-bore tube's other end to the water collection jar.

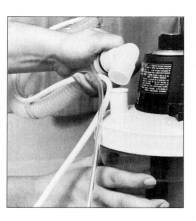

11 In this photo, you'll see the nurse holding the wide-bore tube with the thin tubes attached. Connect the wide-bore tube to the cascade's port.

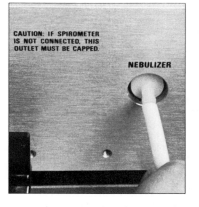

CAUTION: IF SPIROMETER IS NOT CONNECTED, THIS OUTLET MUST BE CAPPED.

NEBULIZER

12 Now, look for the nebulizer valve on the side of the ventilator. Attach the white tube to it.

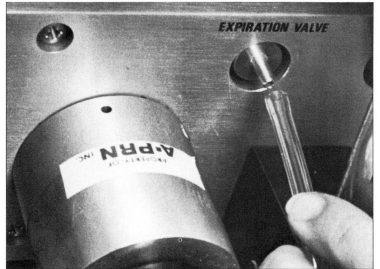

EXPIRATION VALVE

13 On the same side, you'll find the expiration valve. Attach the clear tube to this valve. *Caution:* Check to be sure you've inserted the correct tube in the correct valve. As the photo shows, the expiration valve's on the *left*.

Once you've secured all the tubing and checked the connections for tightness, insert the machine's plug into an electrical outlet. Then, attach the oxygen tube to the wall outlet, and adjust all dials to the prescribed settings. (To better understand ventilator dials, see page 125.) Turn on the ventilator's power switch, and connect the patient.

Ventilators

How to prevent and treat problems caused by mechanical ventilation

Problem	Signs and symptoms	Treatment	Prevention
Pneumothorax, subcutaneous emphysema, or mediastinal emphysema. Usually caused when volume and pressure settings are too high or during administration of PEEP.	With pneumothorax, patient may have absent or diminished breath sounds over affected lung segment, acute pain on affected side, and deviated trachea away from pneumothorax. With subcutaneous emphysema, patient may have crepitus of face, abdomen, and extremities. With mediastinal emphysema, patient shows signs of reduced cardiac output and of crepitus over heart area.	Call doctor immediately; he may insert chest tubes.	Avoid high-pressure settings for high-risk patients; for example, those with COPD, emphysematous blebs, and pulmonary scar tissue.
Atelectasis. Caused by improper deep breathing (sighing), pneumothorax, secretion retention, or a combination of these.	Diminished breath sounds over affected lung segment, decreased compliance; possible change in blood gas values.	Turn patient frequently. Suction and hyperinflate patient's lungs periodically. Use intermittent sighing. The doctor may order bronchoscopy and chest physiotherapy.	Change patient's position frequently. Give chest physiotherapy, and maintain good pulmonary hygiene. Remember to sigh patient frequently.
Cardiovascular impairment. Caused when positive intrathoracic pressure reduces venous return to heart's right side and compresses pulmonary blood circulation.	Decreased blood pressure and cardiac output. Possible decreased urine output. Increased central venous pressure and pulmonary artery pressure.	Doctor may reduce intrathoracic pressure by decreasing PEEP, inspiratory flow rate, and/or tidal volume.	Use PEEP only when necessary. Shorten inspiration time. Maintain adequate blood volume.
Gastrointestinal complications from swallowed air or from stress; for example, GI bleeding, gastric distention, paralytic ileus, and stress ulcer.	Abdominal distention; steady decrease in hemoglobin and hematocrit measurement; positive hematest results on nasogastric drainage and stool; tarry stool.	As ordered, insert nasogastric tube for drainage. Replace lost blood. Use nasogastric tube to give antacids or other medication to decrease acid production.	Avoid giving excessive positive pressure. Reduce patient's psychologic stress. Give antacids and other medications to reduce acid production, with doctor's orders.
Fluid and electrolyte imbalance. Caused by positive water balance.	Probable change in blood gas measurements. Decreased vital capacity, weight gain, ankle edema, moist rales in lungs' lower lobes; pulmonary edema confirmed on X-ray.	Doctor may restrict fluid intake and treat patient for congestive heart failure (if it's present). Rotating tourniquets may be used for pulmonary edema.	Periodically check both blood gas and electrolyte measurements. Monitor patient's fluid intake and ouput. Weigh patient daily.
Tracheal trauma. Caused by constant pressure of cuffed endotracheal tube or nasotracheal tube on the patient's trachea.	Decreased tidal volume from air leak; bleeding from trachea.	Depending on damage, the doctor may insert a trach tube to change position of cuff and allow injured area to heal. Give meticulous cuff care, using minimal leak technique, until tube can be removed.	Give patient proper cuff care, using minimal leak technique when possible. Doctor will use endotracheal or trach tubes with soft cuffs.
Respiratory infection. Caused when upper airway is bypassed, eliminating body's natural defense mechanisms against infection. Also caused by poor aseptic technique.	Elevated temperature and WBC; increased amount, and change in color and odor of respiratory secretions.	Notify doctor. Change patient's position frequently. Perform chest physiotherapy. Use aseptic technique for trach care and for suctioning. Administer prescribed antibiotics.	Maintain good pulmonary hygiene. Use aseptic technique and sterile equipment. Change ventilator tube every 24 hours. Suction patient and hyperinflate his lungs, as needed. Turn patient frequently. Perform chest physiotherapy.
Oxygen toxicity. Caused by excessively high concentrations of oxygen (over 60%) over prolonged period. May cause fibrotic tissue changes in lungs, possibly leading to death.	Burning chest pain on inspiration; dry, hacking cough; dyspnea; decrease in compliance; decreasing PaO_2 on the same oxygen concentration; decreasing vital capacity, and X-ray changes.	Monitor oxygen levels carefully. Report toxicity signs immediately.	Maintain good pulmonary hygiene so low-oxygen concentrations are adequate. Reduce oxygen concentrations as soon as possible.

Ventilator warning signals: What to do

Problem signal	Problem	Possible cause	Nursing intervention
Pressure alarm sounds	Patient's airway obstructed	• Bronchospasm • Patient coughing • Kinked endotracheal tube • Secretion buildup.	• Try to calm patient. • Give bronchodilators as prescribed. • Suction patient. • Straighten tubes and support them with towels. • Suction patient, instilling saline if necessary.
	Patient's fighting ventilator	• Hypoxia • Fear, anxiety • Improvement in patient's condition.	• Obtain and evaluate blood gas measurements. • If blood gas measurements indicate hypoxia, notify doctor so he can adjust percentage of delivered oxygen. • Ask patient if he's getting enough air. *Make sure he's not hypoxic.* • Try to calm patient. Give him writing materials so he can communicate with you. • Give sedation or muscle relaxants, if ordered by doctor. • Begin weaning when ordered by doctor. • Suction patient and hyperinflate his lungs, as needed.
Spirometer alarm sounds	• Power interruption • Leak in delivery system • Leak around trach or endotracheal tube • Spirometer bellows on MA-1 or MA-2 has irregular movement.	• Faulty electrical connection • Disconnected tubing • Nebulizer or cascade humidifier bottles are not screwed on tightly • Torn cuff • Slow leak in cuff • Moisture inside spirometer • Tubing support arm leaning on dipstick, interfering with bellows movement on MA-1 or MA-2.	• Check whether plug's firmly in wall outlet. • Systematically check each connection, beginning with the patient's airway. • Check humidifier or nebulizer bottles to see that they're tightly screwed on. • Deflate cuff and inflate again. If cuff won't seal and patient's still not getting prescribed tidal volume, call the doctor. Hyperinflate patient's lungs until a new tube can be inserted. • Check to see that the spirometer's rubber seal is on tightly. If moisture's inside, dry out spirometer. • Readjust arm so that it clears the dipstick.

Remember: While you're troubleshooting the ventilator, the patient's not getting his prescribed tidal volume. If you can't find the problem source immediately, call for help; begin to hyperinflate the patient's lungs with supplemental oxygen.

___ MINI-ASSESSMENT ___

Weaning: Determining the proper time

How long will your patient need mechanical ventilation? That decision ultimately rests with the doctor. But he'll need your assessment to help him determine when the patient's ready for weaning. To make an accurate assessment, check the patient's condition. Make sure you document all your observations in your nurses' notes.

You'll know your patient's ready if:
• he's awake, has good muscle strength, and has either an adequate natural airway or a functioning tracheostomy.

• he has no life-threatening cardiac arrhythmias and requires little or no vasopressor drugs.
• auscultation and X-ray show that his chest is reasonably clear.
• blood gas analysis shows that his PaO_2 is greater than 60 mm Hg, at a time when he's receiving less than 60% oxygen.
• he can cough effectively enough to mobilize secretions.
• he can generate a reasonable inspiratory force, considering his illness.

Weaning

Weaning your patient from a ventilator

Once the doctor has decided your patient can be weaned from the ventilator, you'll have to prepare him for what's ahead. Before you begin, help set up a weaning schedule that fits into the patient's daily activities. Take care not to schedule weaning periods when the patient may be fatigued from a bath, or an X-ray examination, or immediately after a meal.

Now, talk to the patient. Consider his emotions. If he's been dependent on a ventilator for a long time, he'll probably be scared to leave it. To help alleviate his fears, explain how weaning will help him breathe independently again. Reassure him that you'll watch him carefully and will keep the ventilator nearby in case of trouble.

Prepare the patient physically. Before each weaning period, suction him to clear his airways, and hyperinflate his lungs to expand alveoli. Measure and record his tidal volume, vital capacity, and vital signs. Make sure you have the equipment you'll need to take an arterial blood sample at the bedside.

During the first few weaning periods, stay with your patient and offer encouragement. Record his vital signs every 15 minutes at first, then every half hour, provided he shows signs of successful adjustment. When necessary, suction your patient and hyperinflate his lungs. However, don't do this immediately before you obtain an arterial blood sample. Get the sample first, so you're sure of an accurate blood gas measurement. Watch closely for signs of respiratory distress: labored breathing, restlessness, confusion, blood pressure changes, tremors, or cardiac arrhythmias.

If respiratory distress occurs, obtain a sample of the patient's arterial blood immediately, and send it to the lab for blood gas analysis. Reconnect the patient to the ventilator. Don't wait for a doctor's order to do so; call him afterward. Document the entire episode in your nurses' notes.

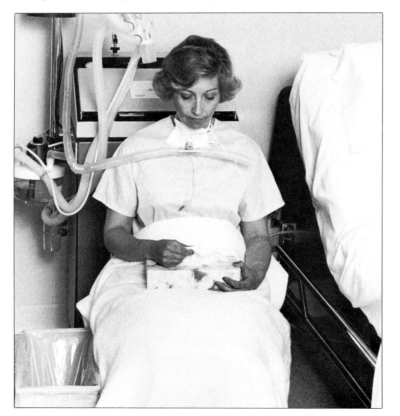

Three ways to wean effectively

Once the doctor's decided that your patient's ready for weaning, he may order one of the following methods. Here's how each works:

Conventional weaning

For this method, first record baseline measurements of your patient's respiratory rate, vital capacity, tidal volume, inspiratory force, heart rate, EKG reading, and blood pressure. Next, disconnect your patient's ventilator, and allow him to breathe spontaneously. At the same time, give him supplemental oxygen and humidity through either a T-piece or a trach collar. After 20 minutes—or sooner, if your patient's condition warrants it—repeat and document the measurements listed above. Then, draw arterial blood for blood gas measurements.

• Continue weaning process if tests show that the patient has satisfactory and stable blood gas measurements, that he has an inspiratory force greater than -20 cm H_2O and that he has a tidal volume of at least 250 ml. *Nursing hint:* Inspiratory force and tidal volume measurements may be less for patients with lung disease.

Over the next 24 to 72 hours, let your patient spend progressively longer periods off the ventilator until he can breathe completely on his own.

• Temporarily discontinue weaning process and reconnect your patient to ventilator if his tests show a significant rise in blood pressure and pulse rate, a progressively decreasing tidal volume, unsatisfactory blood gas measurements, increased fatigue, changed mental status, or the appearance of previously unnoticed cardiac arrhythmias.

Intermittent demand ventilation (IDV)

This method is sometimes called synchronized intermittent mandatory ventilation (SIMV). Don't disconnect your patient's ventilator at first. Instead, set it so it augments his efforts to breathe spontaneously. Then, gradually reduce the number of mechanically assisted breaths per minute. To compensate, your patient will begin increasing his breathing efforts until he eventually can breathe without the ventilator.

While the patient's gaining strength and confidence, offer your encouragement. Carefully monitor his vital capacity, tidal volume, inspiratory force, and vital signs. Periodically draw arterial blood for blood gas measurements.

Intermittent mandatory ventilation (IMV)

With this method, your patient receives a set number of breaths delivered by ventilator during the weaning process. To use it, keep your patient on the ventilator at first, but gradually reduce the frequency of assisted breaths. Continue this process until the patient can breathe on his own. Periodically check patient's vital signs, vital capacity, tidal volume, and inspiratory force. Draw arterial blood for blood gas measurements. Document all findings.

Special nursing considerations

Caring for the patient on a ventilator

Providing good care for the patient on a ventilator requires all your skills and ingenuity. To help you, we offer the following guidelines:

Continue ongoing chest assessments. When you come on duty, check your patient's progress notes for the most recent chest assessment findings. Then, complete your own chest assessment and compare results. Document the details.

Always measure the effectiveness of suctioning and of chest physiotherapy by auscultating your patient's lungs before and after each treatment. For details on how to do this correctly, see Section 1. Record your findings on the patient's progress notes.

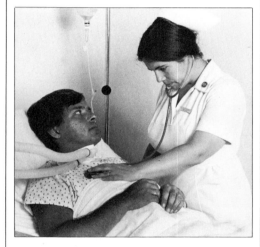

Provide full aeration for your patient's lungs. If the ventilator has a sighing mechanism, set it for hourly deep breathing. If it lacks a sighing mechanism, manually sigh the patient with a hand-held resuscitator six to eight times per hour.

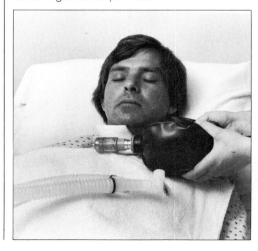

Maintain patient's muscle tone and skin integrity. Turn and reposition your patient at least once every 2 hours. Maintain good body alignment. Remember: Regular turning of your patient also helps prevent atelectasis and pneumonia.

If the doctor orders, perform passive range-of-motion exercises at least once every 4 hours. Turn and position the patient every 2 hours. Encourage him to sit in a bedside chair as much as the doctor orders. If your patient is on a weaning schedule, he may be permitted to walk with assistance. In that case, make sure you have a hand-held resuscitator and a portable oxygen tank handy.

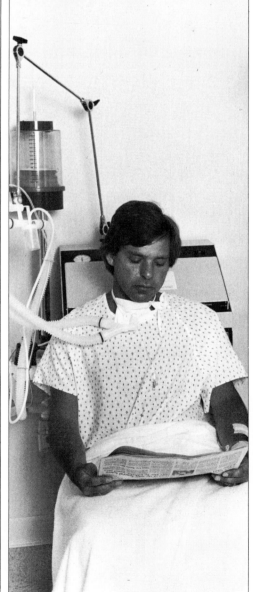

Provide good nutrition and correct fluid and electrolyte balance. Monitor your patient's fluid and electrolyte balance, watching closely for fluid retention, which may indicate a positive water balance.

If he's receiving tube feedings, check for proper tube placement before each meal. Use the correct procedure. Make sure your patient has a diet that's high in carbohydrates and protein.

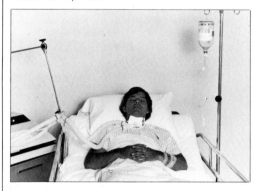

Give your patient a way to communicate. If your patient's conscious, keep writing materials or a Magic Slate at his bedside. Speak to him slowly and clearly, giving him ample time to write his responses. Try to interpret his body language. Watch his facial expressions for signs of anxiety, fear, or discomfort. Take time to explain each procedure before you begin, and give him a chance to write any questions he may have about it. Make sure the call bell's within his reach.

Suppose your patient's comatose. Continue speaking to him, even though he can't answer. Remember, your patient will retain his hearing longer than any of his other senses.

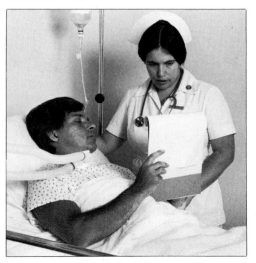

Special nursing considerations

Caring for the patient on a ventilator continued

Keep your patient free of retained secretions. If routine suctioning doesn't remove troublesome secretions, instill 3 to 5 ml of normal saline solution into his endotracheal or tracheostomy tube. Then, hyperinflate his lungs several times with a hand-held resuscitator. Expect him to sputter; then suction him.

Hyperinflate your patient's lungs again after you suction him. Do this by attaching supplemental oxygen to the hand-held resuscitator, or by turning the ventilator's FIO_2 up to 100%. *Caution:* Remember to turn the FIO_2 down to the prescribed rate afterward.

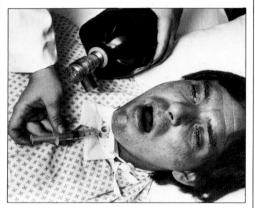

Prevent tracheal damage. To do this, only use endotracheal or tracheostomy tubes with low-pressure cuffs. Provide good cuff care, using the minimal leak technique. For full details on good cuff care, see Section 2.

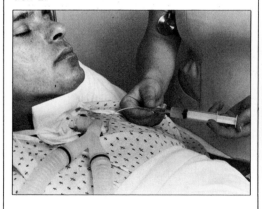

Prevent respiratory tract infection. Wash your hands thoroughly before and after you care for your patient. Use aseptic technique for suctioning. If you notice any change in color, amount, or odor of secretions, obtain a sputum specimen, as explained on page 66.

When you temporarily disconnect the ventilator, for whatever reason, always place the ventilator tube on a sterile towel. Drain the large-bore tube into a wastebasket to remove excess condensation. Take care not to let the tube touch the wastebasket. Empty the ventilator's water collection jar once each shift. Never pour condensation back into cascade.

Make sure the ventilator's working properly and provide humidification. Once each hour, check the ventilator settings for FIO_2, tidal volume, and respiratory rate. Make sure they match the doctor's orders. Keep prescribed settings taped onto the ventilator panel for quick reference. Remember to update them whenever necessary.

As a precaution, in case of ventilator or power failure, place a hand-held resuscitator, oxygen flowmeter, and tubing for supplemental oxygen at the patient's bedside.

For full details on how to properly provide humidification, see Section 3.

Give good eye care. If your patient's receiving a neuromuscular blocking drug like curare or Pavulon, his eyes won't blink or tear. Keep them moist by instilling prescribed eyedrops or washing them with sterile saline solution. To protect them further, close his eyelids and cover them with ¼" nonallergenic tape or oval eye patches.

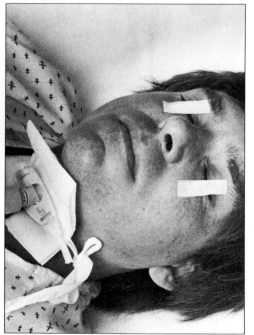

The phrenic pacemaker

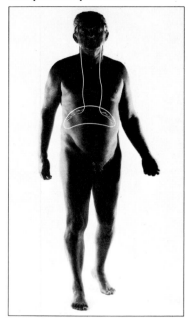

1 When you hear the word pacemaker, what do you think? If you're like most nurses, you immediately think heart. Another kind of pacemaker, though, keeps some patients from long-term dependence on a mechanical ventilator. Called the phrenic, or diaphragm, pacemaker, this respiratory aid helps patients breathe by stimulating the phrenic nerve. Examine the photo to become familiar with this device.

This photo shows the relation of the phrenic nerves to the diaphragm. A diaphragm pacemaker is usually attached to the left phrenic nerve. Why? Because any damage that may occur there will affect pulmonary function less than damage to the right phrenic nerve, which controls ventilation of the larger right lung.

A single pacemaker's usually enough for the patient who has a disease that allows him to breathe on his own while awake. But for the patient who can't, two pacemakers may be necessary, one for each phrenic nerve. In such cases, diaphragm fatigue's prevented by using the two pacemakers alternately, each for no more than 12 hours at a time.

Phrenic nerve pacer

2 The enlarged photo at the right shows the electrode assembly's two ends. A pair of silicone-rubber coated, stainless steel wires join the cuff and twin connectors. To ensure the proper, polarized stimulus, the red-threaded male connector attaches to a similarly threaded female connector on the receiver.

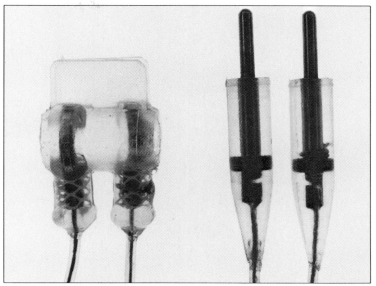

Electrode cuff   Twin connectors

3 The drawing below shows internal placement of the phrenic pacemaker components. The doctor surgically implants an electrode around the phrenic nerve where it crosses the scalenus anticus muscle. Then, he attaches the electrode to a separate subcutaneous receiver.

Once the patient's phrenic nerve's activated, his diaphragm will move. Here's how: A current flows from the transmitter to the antenna, then to the receiver through the electrode connectors, and then to the electrode cuff.

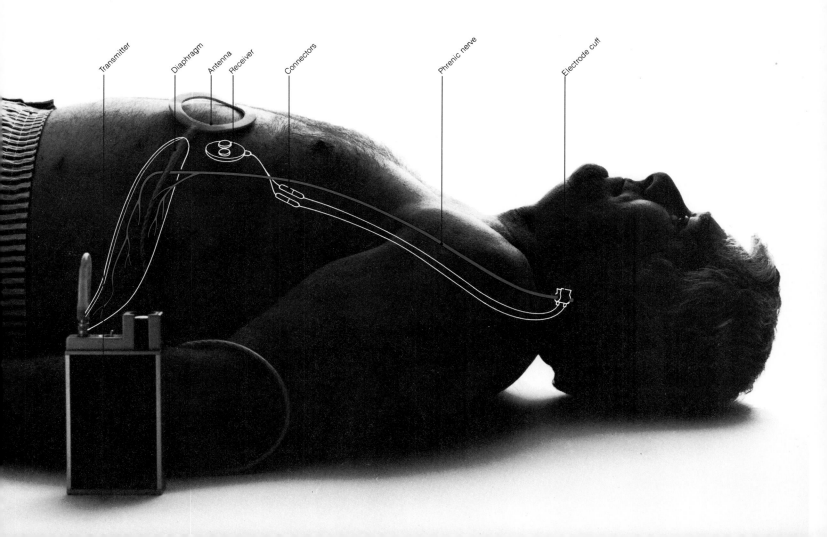

Transmitter   Diaphragm   Antenna   Receiver   Connectors   Phrenic nerve   Electrode cuff

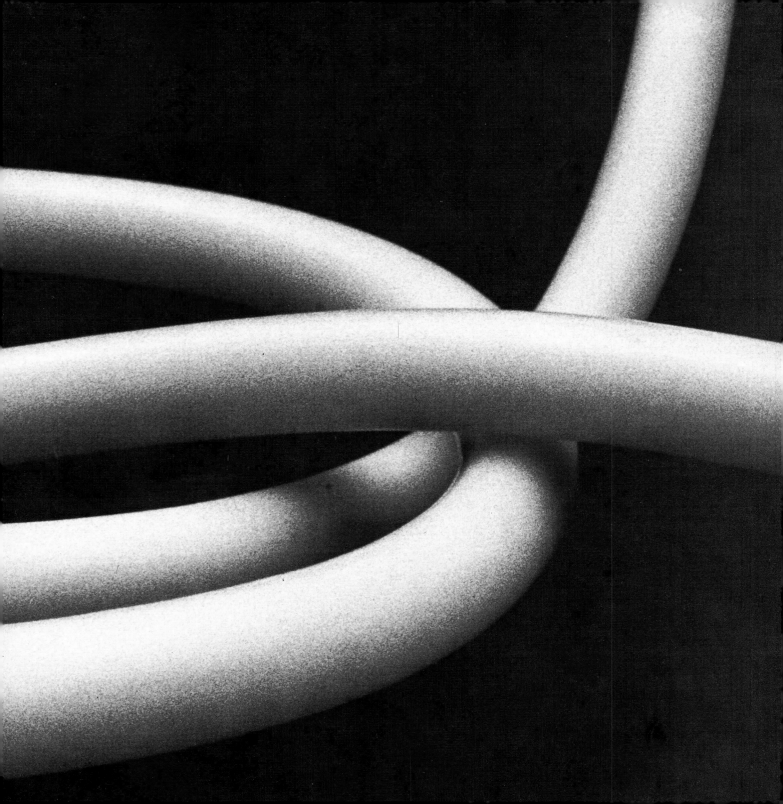

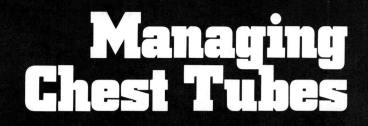

Managing Chest Tubes

Lung pressures
Chest tube insertion
Chest drainage
Chest tube removal
Thoracentesis

Lung pressures

Coping with a patient's chest tubes can be difficult if you're unfamiliar with the complicated procedures and equipment. How well do *you* understand closed chest drainage systems? For example: Do you know how an underwater-seal system works and why it's used?

Can you set up and use a Pleur-evac or Emerson pump? Do you know how to change the drainage system from a one-bottle to a three-bottle setup, if the doctor orders it? Do you know what to do if a patient's chest tube gets disconnected?

On the following pages, we'll answer all these questions. Then you can care for patients with chest drainage confidently and intelligently.

A quick review of basic terms

To better understand what we're talking about when we explain chest drainage systems, review the definitions of these terms:

Atmospheric pressure: The pressure exerted by the atmosphere: 760 mm Hg at sea level.
Positive pressure: A pressure greater than atmospheric pressure. It exerts a blowing force.
Negative pressure: A pressure less than atmospheric pressure. It exerts a pulling force.

Parietal pleura: The thin membrane that lines the chest cavity.
Visceral pleura: The thin membrane lining lungs.
Pleural cavity: The potential space between the visceral and the parietal pleurae.
Pneumothorax: An accumulation of air in the pleural cavity, which causes lung collapse.
Hemothorax: An accumulation of bloody fluid in the pleural cavity, which causes lung collapse.

How normal pressures affect the resting lung

Atmospheric pressure
760 mm Hg

Intrapulmonary pressure
760 mm Hg

Lung elasticity
−5 cm H₂O

Parietal pleura

Visceral pleura

Pleural cavity

Bronchus

Intrapleural pressure
755 mm Hg

1 *Above, you'll see an illustration of the normal lung at rest.* As you know, lungs contain a large amount of elastic tissue, which is constantly trying to contract (like a stretched rubber band). However, negative pressure within the pleural cavity exerts a suctioning force on the lungs, preventing collapse. The lungs' natural elastic recoil produces intrapleural negative pressures of −5 cm at rest; −6 to −12 cm water during inspiration; and −4 to −8 cm water during expiration.

2 Pressure differences also affect the bellows-like movement of air into and out of the lungs. To understand how, remember this rule—*all gases move from a place of greater pressure to a place of lesser pressure.*

Here you see an illustration of a normal chest in the resting phase. Because no difference exists in pressures between the outside air and the lungs, no air moves. The lungs will not collapse because of intrapleural negative pressure.

3 On inspiration, the diaphragm contracts and the chest cavity enlarges. The intrapleural negative pressure drops, pulling the lungs close to the ribs. This enlarges lung space, causing its pressure to fall below the atmospheric pressure, although *not* below the intrapleural negative pressure. According to the rule we just stated, air enters the lungs. (To better understand the physiologic changes that we've described here, study the arrows and symbols in this illustration.)

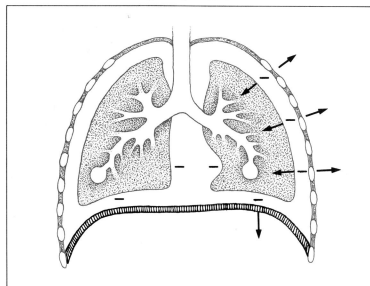

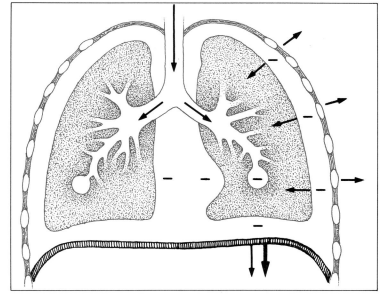

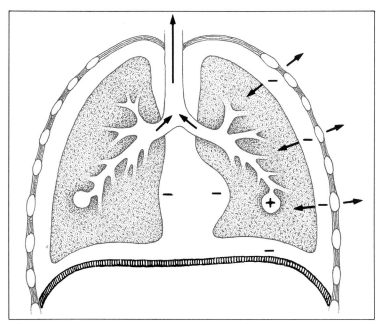

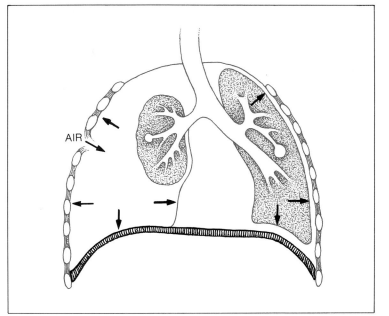

4 On expiration, the diaphragm recoils and the chest cavity shrinks. Intrapleural pressure rises, although it remains negative. As the lungs are compressed, their pressure rises above atmospheric pressure. According to the rule stated before, air moves out of the lungs into the atmosphere. (To better understand physiologic changes that occur on expiration, study this illustration and compare the arrows and symbols for inspiration.)

5 If injury or surgery causes a large amount of air to enter the pleural cavity, negative pressure is lost. The suctioning force on each lung is weakened. Nothing prevents the lungs' elastic tissue from contracting, and the lungs collapse.

Important: Any fluid that collects in the pleural cavity can also collapse the lungs, because it takes up the space the lungs need to expand.

Chest tube insertion

Indications for chest tube insertion

Problem	Cause	Signs and symptoms
Hemothorax (blood in pleural space)	• Trauma to chest wall, lung tissue, or mediastinum • Pulmonary infarction • Pleural or pulmonary neoplasm • Pleural tear, resulting from spontaneous pneumothorax • Complication of anticoagulant therapy following chest surgery.	Your patient may have any of these signs and symptoms. Remember, however, that in some cases, hemothorax is asymptomatic. In other cases, the patient may exhibit signs of profound circulatory collapse. • Shock, tachycardia, diaphoresis, hypotension, skin color changes • Chest pain • Dyspnea • Asymmetric chest movements, if hemothorax is large • Diminished or absent breath sounds on affected side • Dullness on percussion.
Pneumothorax (air in pleural space)	• Blunt chest trauma caused by a fall, blow, violent cough, or sudden deceleration. *Note:* In deceleration injuries, the lungs may be thrown forward, causing a pleural tear or severe laceration of the bronchi, with resultant lung collapse and hemorrhage. • Penetrating chest injury, such as a knife or bullet wound • Complication of thoracentesis.	Your patient may have any of these signs and symptoms. Remember, they may vary according to the size of the pneumothorax. • Sudden sharp chest pain, which may be referred to corresponding shoulder, across chest, or abdomen • Dyspnea • Dry, hacking cough • Asymmetric chest movements • Diminished or absent breath sounds on affected side • Hyperresonance on percussion • Subcutaneous emphysema around neck (in some cases).
Spontaneous pneumothorax (air in pleural space without apparent cause)	• Chronic lung disorders, such as emphysema, in which a subpleural cyst, bulla, or bleb ruptures. Endomorphic patients commonly have congenital blebs.	• Sudden sharp chest pain, which may be referred to corresponding shoulder, across chest, or abdomen • Dyspnea • Dry, hacking cough • Asymmetric chest movements • Diminished or absent breath sounds on affected side • Hyperresonance on percussion • Subcutaneous emphysema around neck (in some cases).
Tension pneumothorax (air enters pleural space with each inspiration and becomes trapped, causing pressure buildup as it accumulates)	• Puncture wound to the chest • Mechanical ventilators, especially when delivering PEEP, may rupture a bleb. • Faulty underwater-seal drainage system • Prolonged clamping of chest tube.	• Severe dyspnea • Marked cyanosis • Tachycardia • Shift of mediastinum to unaffected side • Diminished or absent tactile fremitus • Hyperresonance on percussion.
Mediastinal shift	• Severe tension pneumothorax. *Notify the doctor immediately.* Such a patient needs prompt medical attention to save his life.	• Deviation of larynx and trachea from midline toward unaffected side • Percussion reveals displacement of cardiac dullness. On auscultation, the apex beat is shifted. • Cardiac arrhythmias • If cardiac output is drastically diminished, patient has distended neck veins, and negligible blood pressure.
Hemopneumothorax (air and blood in pleural space, with possible clotting)	• Blunt or penetrating chest wound • Complication of chest surgery.	Same as for hemothorax and pneumothorax.

Closed chest drainage: How it helps

When your patient needs it, the doctor may choose closed chest drainage, sometimes called the underwater-seal method, to accomplish one or more of the following:
• remove accumulated liquids, such as blood, pus, chyle, serous fluids, or gastric juices, from his pleural space
• remove accumulated air from his pleural space
• remove solids, such as clotted blood fibrin, from the patient's pleural space
• restore negative pressure to his pleural space
• reexpand a collapsed or partially collapsed lung.

How to position your patient for chest tube insertion

1 *If your patient has a collapsed lung, for whatever reason, the doctor may want to insert a chest tube and may ask you to assist. Will you know how to properly position your patient? Follow these guidelines, remembering that the cause of the collapsed lung dictates where the tube's inserted.*

Suppose, for example, your patient has a pneumothorax and needs a chest tube to remove accumulated air from his pleural cavity. To prepare him, place him flat on his back. The doctor will probably insert an apical tube in the second or third intercostal space of the patient's chest.

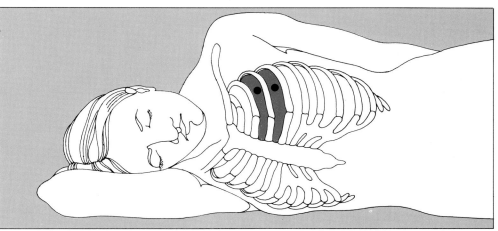

2 If your patient has a hemothorax, he may need a chest tube to remove accumulated blood from his pleural cavity. Prepare him by placing him on his back, and elevate the bed to a semi-Fowler's position. The doctor will probably insert a basilar tube in the sixth or seventh intercostal space along the midaxillary line.

Important: If your patient can't tolerate an elevated position, place him on his side, with his affected side up.

3 Has your patient just had a thoracotomy? Does he have blood *and* air in his pleural cavity? The doctor will want to insert two chest tubes: a basilar and an apical. In that case, place the patient on his back in the appropriate position (see above description). The doctor will then insert the tubes, as we already explained.

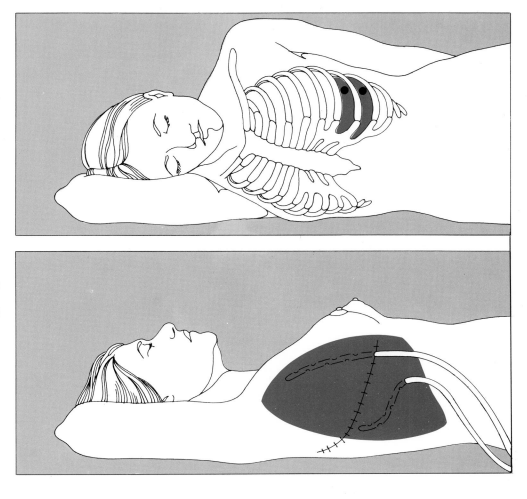

Chest drainage

How to make a flutter valve

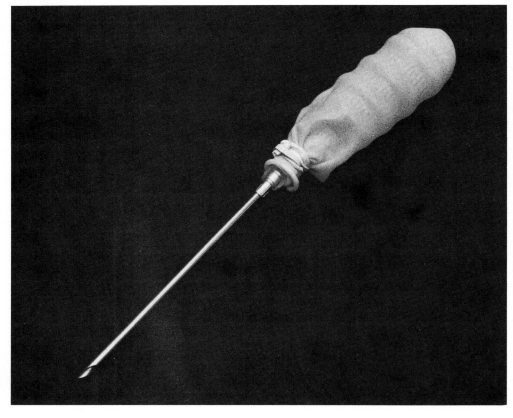

Suppose your patient develops a tension pneumothorax. To prevent a life-threatening mediastinal shift, the doctor may insert a flutter valve.

This improvised emergency device allows trapped air to escape from the lungs during expiration, without allowing room air to enter through the valve during inspiration. The necessary equipment, already assembled, is pictured here: a large-bore (12G or 14G) needle, a finger cot that's been perforated with a pin, and a small rubber band.

When you've gathered the necessary equipment, the doctor will first insert the large-bore needle into the affected pleural space. Then, he'll attach the finger cot to the needle hub, with a rubber band. *Remember:* The flutter valve's only a temporary solution to a tension pneumothorax. Be prepared to assist the doctor as he inserts chest tube.

Underwater-seal chest drainage: How it works

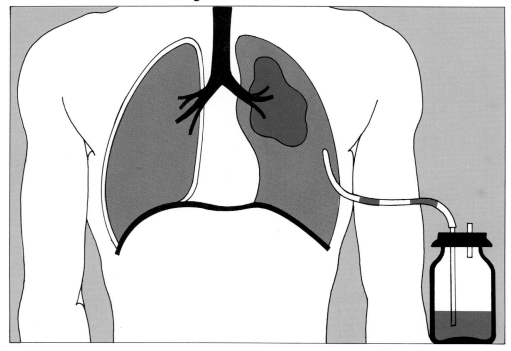

Confused about the basic principle behind underwater-seal chest drainage? This illustration will help you. To use this method, the doctor first inserts a chest tube into the patient's pleural cavity. Then, he connects the chest tube to the tube extending to the long glass straw in the drainage bottle. Notice how the end of the glass straw is always kept underwater. This prevents drained air or fluid from backing up the tube into the patient's pleural cavity. The short glass tube on the bottle acts as an air vent.

Getting acquainted with the Pleur-evac

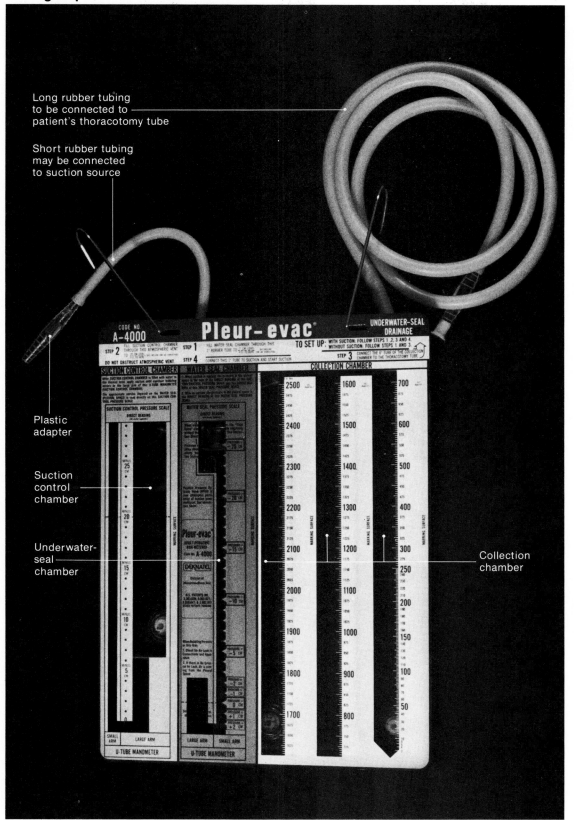

Long rubber tubing to be connected to patient's thoracotomy tube

Short rubber tubing may be connected to suction source

Plastic adapter

Suction control chamber

Underwater-seal chamber

Collection chamber

To save time and eliminate the risk of bottle breakage, many hospitals now use disposable underwater-seal chest drainage systems. The Pleur-evac, which is one such system, is illustrated here. As you can see, it has the basic three-bottle setup enclosed in one unit. The instructions and measurements printed on the front of the unit make it easy to use.

Chest drainage

How to set up and use a Pleur-evac

1 *Picture yourself in this situation. The doctor decides your patient needs a chest tube inserted and wants you to assist. What must you do?* First, make sure the patient's signed the surgical consent form. Answer any questions he may have. Then, gather the equipment the doctor will need (including a suction device), and obtain a disposable Pleur-evac. Unwrap the Pleur-evac carefully, and hang it on its disposable floor stand. Or hang it from the bedframe. To fill it, you'll need a large container of sterile water and a 60 ml piston or bulb syringe.

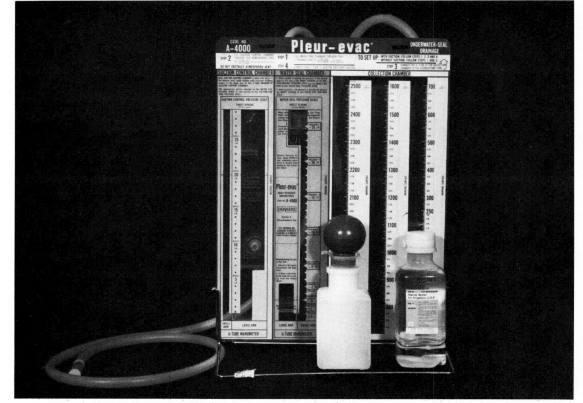

2 Now, remove the plastic connector on the short tube attached to the water-seal chamber. Remove the plunger or bulb from the syringe and attach barrel. Pour water into the tube, using the syringe barrel as a funnel.

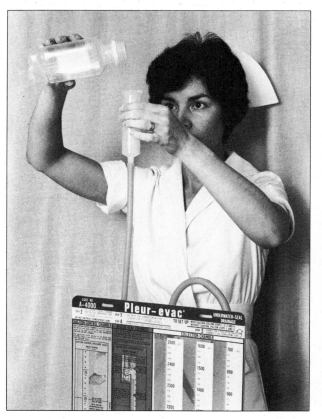

3 Always fill the water-seal chamber to the 2 cm level no matter what the doctor decides to do about suctioning. Remember to check the water level periodically. Refill the chamber, as needed.

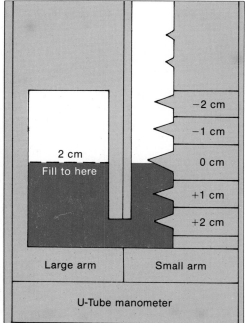

4 If the doctor doesn't want suction used, leave the end of this short tube unclamped. This will allow air to escape from the pleural cavity.

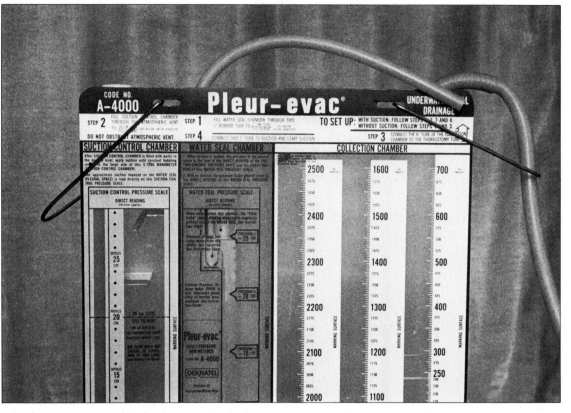

5 If the doctor does want suction used, remove the plastic muffler from the vent to the suction control chamber. Attach a syringe barrel to the vent, using the same method as before, and pour water into the chamber.

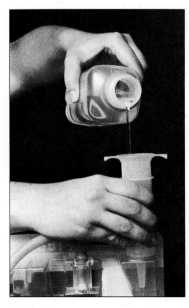

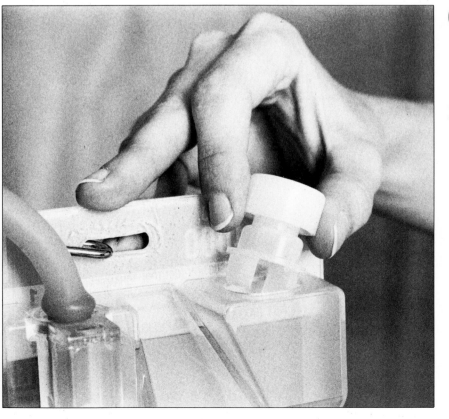

6 Fill the suction control chamber to the 20 cm level, or as ordered. Replace the plastic muffler to minimize bubbling noise. *Make sure nothing occludes the vent.*
Important: Always check the water level in the suction chamber at least once each shift. If evaporation occurs, you'll have to refill the chamber.

Chest drainage

How to set up and use a Pleur-evac continued

7 At this point, the doctor will prepare the patient and insert the chest tube, with your assistance. When he does, remove the adapter from the long tube that extends from the Pleur-evac's collection chamber. Stand by as the doctor connects this tube to the patient's chest tube. Tape over the connections to prevent air leaks and to keep tubes securely together. However, never completely occlude the plastic connector. You must observe drainage.

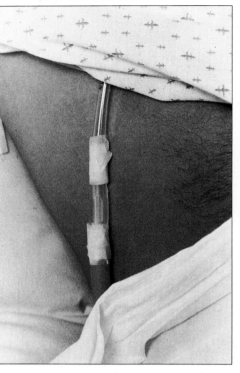

8 Has the doctor ordered suction? Connect the short tube on the water-seal chamber to the suction device, using the plastic connector provided. Turn on the suction and slowly increase it until bubbling occurs in the suction control chamber.

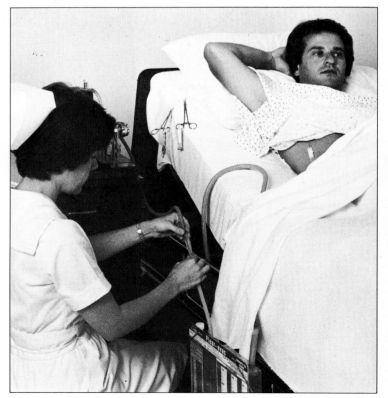

9 At the end of each shift, measure the drainage that has accumulated in the collection chamber. Indicate on the front of the unit the date and hour you measured it. *Important:* When you measure drainage, remember to read at eye level.

Here's another important reminder: Spillover from one chamber to the next may occur, especially if the unit's moved. This may decrease the volume you previously noted in the first chamber. To avoid error, check the volume of each chamber before you total the output.

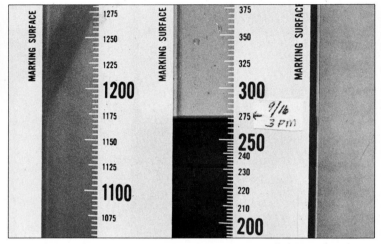

10 You may need a specimen of chest drainage so it can be analyzed. To obtain it, attach a syringe with 18G or 20G needle to the self-sealing diaphragm in back of the collection chamber. Withdraw the desired amount, cap and label the syringe, and send it to the lab. Make sure the needle's securely attached.

Important: Never attempt to empty entire contents of collection chamber through this diaphragm. If collection chamber completely fills, the whole unit must be replaced.

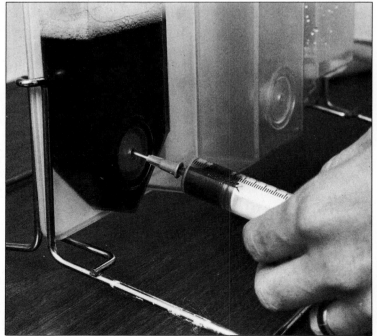

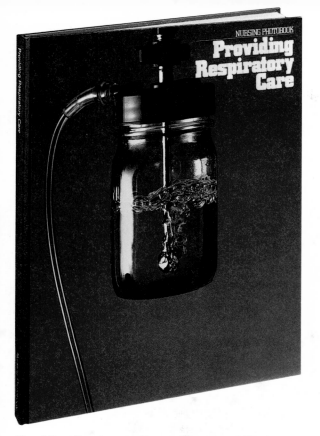

Providing Respiratory Care will answer all your questions about airway obstruction and respiratory inadequacy. And it will introduce you to the NURSING PHOTOBOOK series, the all-new reference books from the publishers of *NURSING79* and the NURSING SKILLBOOK series.

To examine *Providing Respiratory Care* for 10 days without cost or obligation, return the attached order card today. And find out what you can do to overcome your patients' breathing difficulties.

Send for *Providing Respiratory Care* today and see how the PHOTOBOOK series can make you a better nurse

This illustrated nursing guide shows—and tells—you everything you need to know about providing respiratory care. Sharp, clear photographs and drawings are supplemented by authoritative text. So you can see for yourself the most professional way to position your patient for chest tube insertions • Avoid—or solve—suctioning problems • Set up an Emerson pump • Teach home trach care • Understand mechanical ventilator cycles • Draw arterial blood for blood gas measurements • Convert a non-rebreathing mask to a partial rebreather • And more.

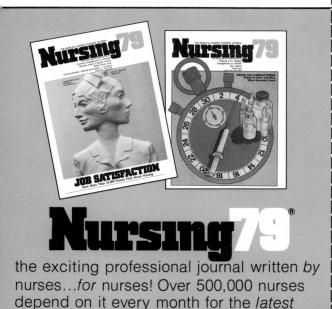

the exciting professional journal written *by* nurses...*for* nurses! Over 500,000 nurses depend on it every month for the *latest* clinical information on direct patient care.

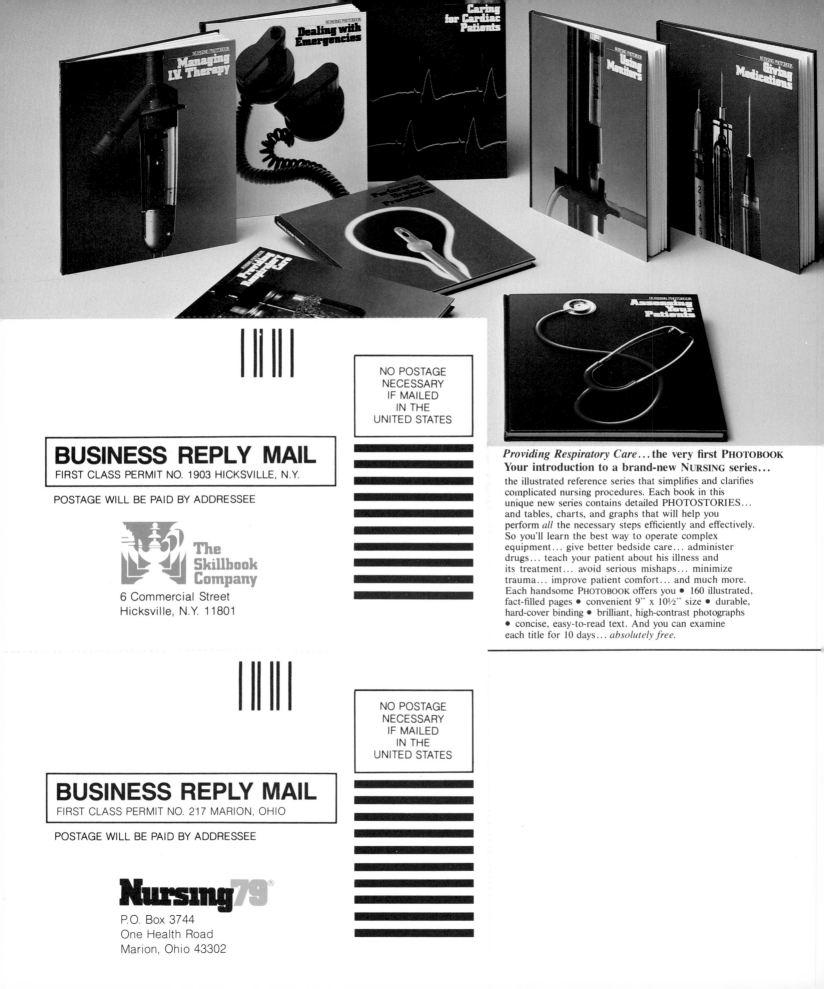

Providing Respiratory Care... the very first PHOTOBOOK
Your introduction to a brand-new NURSING series...

the illustrated reference series that simplifies and clarifies complicated nursing procedures. Each book in this unique new series contains detailed PHOTOSTORIES... and tables, charts, and graphs that will help you perform *all* the necessary steps efficiently and effectively. So you'll learn the best way to operate complex equipment... give better bedside care... administer drugs... teach your patient about his illness and its treatment... avoid serious mishaps... minimize trauma... improve patient comfort... and much more. Each handsome PHOTOBOOK offers you ● 160 illustrated, fact-filled pages ● convenient 9" x 10½" size ● durable, hard-cover binding ● brilliant, high-contrast photographs ● concise, easy-to-read text. And you can examine each title for 10 days... *absolutely free.*

Using the one-bottle setup

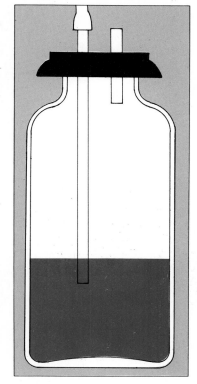

Your hospital may still use a glass bottle chest drainage system. If so, you're probably familiar with the one-, two-, and three-bottle setups. In this photostory, we're explaining how to use the one-bottle setup for straight gravity drainage.

Unwrap and assemble it, making sure you maintain sterility. Then, prepare your patient for chest tube insertion, as explained on page 139.

Now, study this illustration. As you can see, the bottle serves as both the collection receptacle and the underwater-seal chamber. To set it up properly, pour sterile water into the bottle until the end of the long glass straw is submerged 2 cm. Connect the straw to the drainage tube, maintaining strict sterility.

Assist the doctor as he inserts the chest tube. After he does, connect the chest tube to the drainage tube.

Important: Always keep the short glass straw uncovered so it can act as an air vent. If you cover it, you'll prevent air from escaping from your patient's pleural cavity.

How to use suction with a nondisposable underwater-seal chest drainage

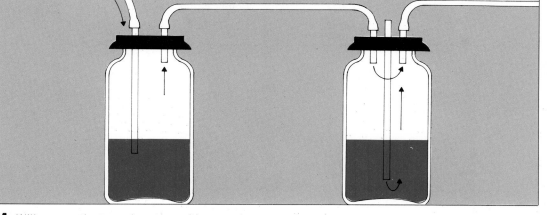

1 *Will your patient need suction with an underwater-seal chest drainage system? The doctor will decide. He may order it from the start or add it later if a chest X-ray confirms that the patient's lung isn't reexpanding. If he does, he'll probably specify the two-bottle setup shown in this illustration. Here's how to assemble it:*

First, prepare the straight gravity drainage bottle as explained earlier. Then, prepare the suction control bottle like this: Run a tube from the air vent on the drainage bottle to one of the short glass straws on the suction control bottle. Then, insert a long glass straw in the middle of the suction control bottle. Run a tube from the remaining short glass straw on that bottle to the suction equipment. Never cover the long glass straw; it's an air vent. Get ready to fill the suction control bottle with sterile water. But first, find out from the doctor how much suction the patient should receive. The amount of suction (or negative pressure) is regulated by the distance between the water surface and the submerged end of the long glass straw. (Usual distance ordered is 10 cm to 20 cm.) Fill bottle as directed.

If the prescribed amount of suction is ineffective, the doctor may ask you to add more sterile water to increase it. Or he may order controlled suction delivered by an Emerson pump (see page 146).

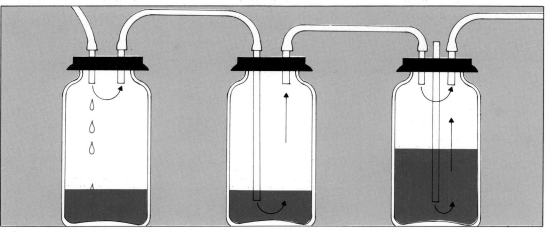

2 In some cases, the doctor may prefer a three-bottle setup when he wants suction. To see how this works, examine this illustration. As you can see, this setup has a separate collection bottle. No matter which setup you use, follow these guidelines:
• Always place glass bottles in a heavy wire floor rack to prevent breakage. Never place bottles under the patient's bed.
• Keep bottles lower than the patient's chest at all times.
• If the underwater-seal bottle is accidentally broken, immediately clamp the patient's chest tube close to his chest. Work quickly to replace the bottle. Remember, when the chest tube is clamped, the air or fluid that's accumulating in his pleural cavity has no way to escape. For details on clamping chest tubes, see page 148.
• Anytime a large amount of drainage accumulates in the underwater-seal bottle, negative pressure increases, making it difficult for air and fluid to escape from the patient's pleural cavity. If this happens, the doctor may want the bottle changed. Remember to clamp the tube first.

Chest drainage

Setting up the Emerson pleural suction pump

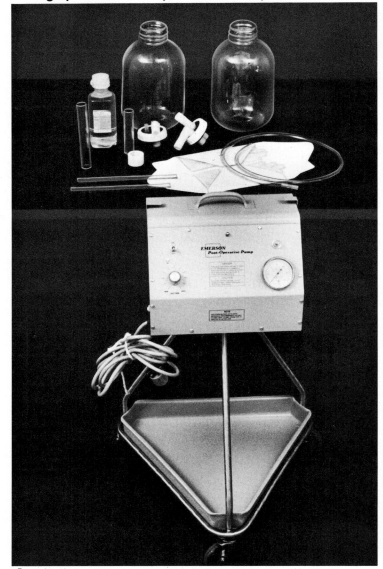

1 *Does your patient have a large amount of air or fluid in his pleural space? To remove it efficiently, the doctor may wish to connect his chest tube to an Emerson pleural suction pump. Because it's adjustable, the Emerson pump allows you to control exactly how much negative pressure your patient's receiving. What's more, if the patient's tubing becomes obstructed, a built-in safety feature keeps the pump from climbing to dangerously high negative pressures.*

Here's how to set it up: First, gather the necessary equipment. Besides the pump itself, you'll need a primary trap bottle with a three-connector cap; a secondary trap bottle with a two-connector cap; two plastic straws, 9½" long x ⅜" in diameter; one or two long drainage tubes with connectors (depending on how many catheters your patient has); two wide-bore connector tubes, 4½" and 6½"; sterile gloves; sterile water; and adhesive tape.

Second, check to see if the pump's functioning. Plug it into the nearest electric outlet, turn on the on/off switch, and note whether the red indicator light goes on. Turn off the pump, making sure that the pressure control knob's turned down to just below minimal.

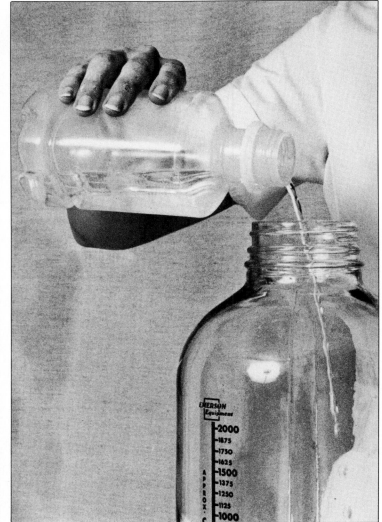

2 Now, unwrap all the other equipment, leaving the sterile wrappers underneath. Take the primary trap bottle, which has graduated markings, and fill it with sterile water up to the water line.

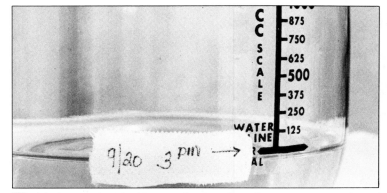

3 Mark water level with an adhesive strip. For greater precision, draw an arrow pointing to the exact level. Be sure to indicate date and time. Later, you'll use additional adhesive strips at prescribed intervals to show drainage volume.

4 Put on the sterile gloves. Then, pick up the primary trap bottle's cap, which has three connectors—one wide and two narrow—and connect both plastic straws to its underside, as shown in this photo. Secure the cap tightly. *Important:* Make sure the straws project 1" below the water's surface, to create a proper seal.

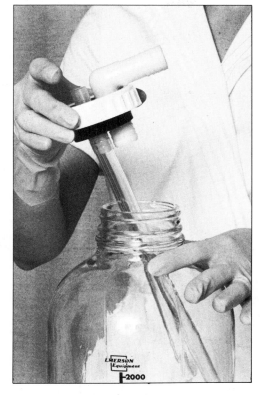

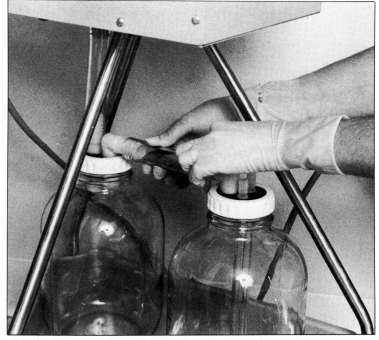

7 Next, place the primary trap bottle on the shelf, and connect it to the secondary trap bottle with the 4½" wide-bore connector tube. Again, check for tightness.

5 Next, screw the cap on the secondary trap bottle, as the nurse is doing in the photo opposite.

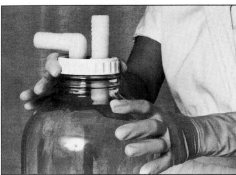

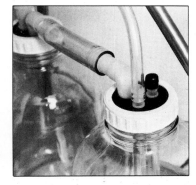

8 Attach the long chest drainage tubes to the connectors on the primary trap bottle's cap. If your patient's going to have only one chest tube, use just one drainage tube and cap the other connector. Until the doctor connects the drainage tube to the catheter, keep the drainage tube's free end capped or covered to maintain sterility.

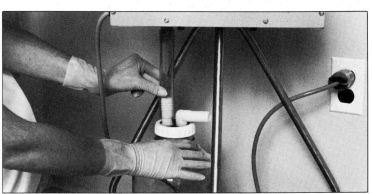

6 Place the secondary trap bottle on the Emerson pump's lower shelf. This bottle acts as a reserve, in case of frothy overflow. Use the 6½" wide-bore connector tube to attach it to the pump. Check all connections for tightness.

9 After the doctor has inserted the chest tube, he'll use a connector to attach it to the long drainage tube. Now the pump's ready for use. At the doctor's order, turn on the machine. Slowly adjust the pressure control knob until the gauge registers the prescribed pressure. Usually, this'll be −20 cm H_2O, although in some cases it may be as high as −60. To prevent tampering, you may be asked to place adhesive tape over the pressure control knob once the correct pressure is reached.

Chest drainage

Coping with chest tubes: Questions nurses ask

If you're like most nurses, you probably have lots of questions about chest tube management. On the following pages, we've supplied answers to some of those questions, so you can properly care for your patient and cope with any problems that occur.

What's the greatest risk for a patient with chest tubes? How can I prevent it?

When a patient has one or more chest tubes, he risks a tension pneumothorax from accumulated air or fluid in his pleural cavity. Prevent it by following these guidelines:
• Keep the underwater-seal drainage system properly vented so air can escape from the pleural cavity.
• Use precautions to prevent bottle breakage.
• Take care not to accidentally disconnect tubes.
• Never clamp a chest tube unless it's absolutely necessary. If you must, keep it clamped for only a brief period.

How can I tell if the underwater-seal drainage system is working properly?

Chances are, it is if your patient shows no evidence of respiratory distress. But look for the following signs indicating all's well:
• Moderate bubbling in suction control chamber of Pleur-evac or bottle system (if patient's getting suction).
• Moderate bubbling in underwater-seal chamber of Pleur-evac or bottle system (if patient has pneumothorax).
• Water-level fluctuation in underwater-seal chamber of Pleur-evac or bottle system as patient inhales and exhales.

What should I do if the bubbling in the suction control chamber stops?

Check the tubes for possible air leaks. If no air leak exists, call the doctor. He may want you to increase suction.

What should I do if bubbling becomes excessive in the underwater-seal chamber of Pleur-evac or bottle system?

Excessive bubbling may indicate an air leak in the tubes outside or within the patient's chest cavity. Call the doctor.

To discover the leak's location, the doctor may ask you to first clamp the chest tube close to the patient's chest. If the bubbling stops, the leak's located within the chest cavity or at the insertion site.

Suppose the bubbling doesn't stop. The doctor may then ask you to clamp the drainage tube at points further along the tube. If he does, work your way down the tube until you discover the leak. Then, tape the loose connection or replace the drainage tube.

Important: Never replace a drainage tube without first clamping the chest tube.

What should I do if water-level fluctuations in the underwater-seal chamber cease?

Check all tubes. Make sure they aren't kinked, looped, or wedged underneath the patient. Look for clots inside the tubes. Instruct your patient to cough and to change his position. This may dislodge a small obstruction in the tube. Check the suction apparatus to make sure it's working properly.

If none of these measures helps, call the doctor. Remember: Cessation of water-level fluctuations may mean your patient's lung has reexpanded and no longer requires chest drainage.

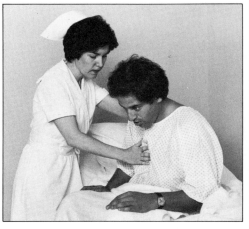

Under what circumstances should I clamp my patient's chest tubes?

Do it immediately if a glass underwater-seal bottle breaks. However, in the following situations, let the doctor make the decision:
• If the drainage bottle or Pleur-evac becomes full and needs replacing.
• If you need to collect a drainage specimen from the bottle.
• If your patient's being transported with glass bottles, increasing the risk of breakage.
• If your patient's condition has so improved that he no longer needs a chest tube. In such a case, the doctor may want to clamp before removal, to test the patient's reaction.

How do I clamp a chest tube?

Using a covered Kelly clamp, clamp the tube about 10 inches from the insertion site. To make sure it's secure, apply a second clamp pointed in the opposite direction.

Never use a metal clamp, because it may damage the tube. Always keep two covered clamps at the patient's bedside for emergency use. Clamp them to the bed linen (near the headboard), so you can find them quickly.

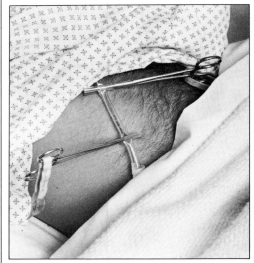

How can I prevent complications in a patient with chest tubes?

Vary your patient's position regularly to keep him from retaining secretions. But check with the doctor first to see which positions to avoid. Place the patient in semi-Fowler's position to permit accumulated air to rise and escape through the chest tube. Your patient will find it easier to breathe in this position.

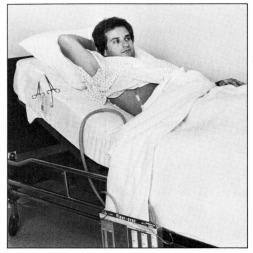

Turn him every 2 hours. Make sure the tubes don't kink or loop during turning. Keep them secure so they don't become accidentally disconnected.

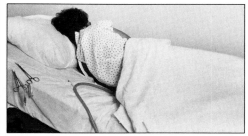

Teach the patient range-of-motion exercises for the arm on his affected side. These exercises will help prevent ankylosis. Make sure your patient coughs and deep breathes hourly, preferably in a sitting position. Show him how to splint the tube's insertion site. Help him with splinting, if necessary.

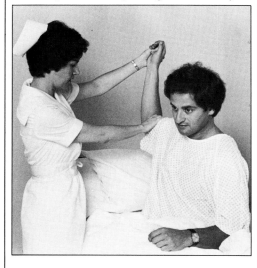

Suppose a patient with chest tubes has to be transported by stretcher.
Make sure the Pleur-evac or drainage bottles stay below the patient's chest level. If he has a Pleur-evac with suction, disconnect the tube leading to the suction apparatus. Leave it unclamped, so it can act as an air vent.

If your patient has a glass-bottle chest drainage system, bottle breakage may occur during transport. Ask the doctor if he wants you to clamp the patient's chest tubes as a precaution against this emergency. But make sure the clamps are removed when the patient reaches his destination.

If the doctor doesn't want the chest tubes clamped, take even greater care to make sure the bottles don't get broken. Inform others how and when to clamp tubes.

How can I prevent clots from obstructing the drainage tube?
If your patient has bloody drainage from a hemothorax or thoracotomy, the doctor may want you to strip the drainage tube every 30 minutes to every 2 hours, depending on the drainage. Here's how:

Start at the top end of the drainage tube. With one hand, compress the top end tightly, allowing slack to keep from pulling on the chest tube's insertion site. With your other hand, flatten the drainage tube between your thumb and index finger, and slide your hand down the full length of the tube. Without releasing pressure, strip drainage into the collection chamber.

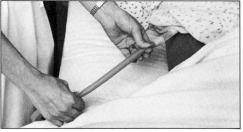

You may also use a mechanical stripper for this procedure. The one shown below was devised by a nurse in Florida.

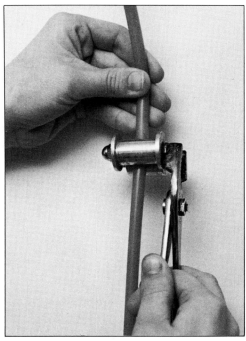

What do I do if my patient's chest tube gets accidentally disconnected from the drainage tube?
Reconnect it immediately. If you can't because you've lost or broken a connector,

clamp the chest tube until you've remedied the problem. Work quickly so you can reconnect the tube as soon as possible. Remember to unclamp the chest tube when you've completed the connection.

What do I do if my patient's chest tube falls out or is accidentally pulled out?
Quickly seal off the insertion site to prevent air from entering his pleural cavity. Use Vaseline gauze and cover it with 4" x 4" gauze pads. Tape securely. If gauze isn't handy, temporarily seal the insertion site with a folded towel. Call the doctor immediately. Ask another nurse to get the equipment the doctor will need to reinsert the tubes.

Don't leave the patient. Watch him for signs of pneumothorax, as described on page 138. Tension pneumothorax may occur because you've sealed off the only escape route for accumulating air or fluid. If danger signs do appear, remove the dressings immediately.

What observations should I make about chest drainage and how should I document them?
Observe the amount, color, and consistency of chest drainage by looking through the plastic connector between the chest tube and the drainage tube.

Check it hourly for the first 24 hours after chest tube insertion; then once every 2 hours. Document your findings.

At no time should bloody drainage exceed 100 ml per hour, even after chest surgery. If it does, notify the doctor at once. If drainage decreases or stops altogether, check for problems in the tube. Remember, however, that it may indicate the patient's condition is improving.

Keep the label on the drainage bottle up to date. Always write the amount of drainage that your patient's had over an 8-hour shift.

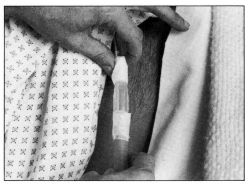

Chest tube removal

Assisting the doctor with chest tube removal

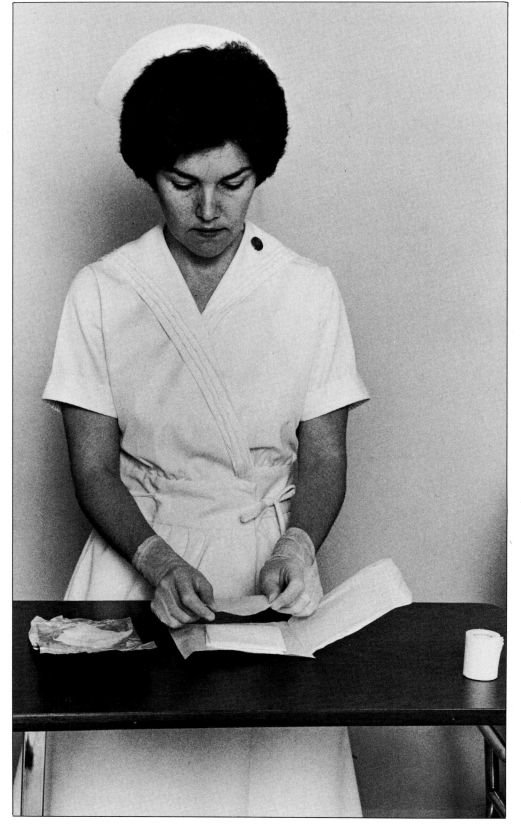

1 *Your patient's chest X-ray shows a fully reexpanded lung, and the doctor's going to remove the chest tube.* To help, gather the following equipment: sterile gloves; three or four sterile 4" x 4" gauze pads; sterile Vaseline gauze; sterile suture removal kit; bedsaver pad; and 2"- to 3"-wide adhesive tape.

Place the patient in semi-Fowler's position. As the doctor explains the procedure to the patient, prepare the necessary materials. Here's how: First, lay the bedsaver pad next to patient, partially against his chest. Open the packages of gauze pads and of Vaseline gauze. Open the suture removal kit. Then, slip on sterile gloves. Pick up the Vaseline gauze and place it over the 4" x 4" gauze pads, as the nurse is doing here.

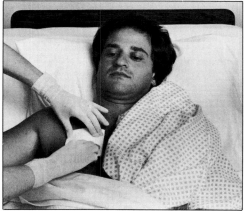

2 The doctor will begin the procedure by clamping the chest tube. Then, he'll remove the suture provided it's not the purse-string type. Next, he'll loosen the dressing and move it away from the insertion site. Then, he'll slip on sterile gloves to complete the procedure. Next, he'll take the sterile dressing or ask you to place it over (but not touching) the insertion site. The doctor will then instruct the patient to inhale deeply and hold his breath as the tube is quickly removed. This prevents air from being sucked into the patient's chest.

Once the tube's out, the sterile dressing must be quickly put over the insertion site, as shown here. Make sure the Vaseline gauze is against the skin. Secure the pads with adhesive tape, to prevent an air leak. *Note:* If the patient has a purse-string suture, the doctor will pull it closed and tie it tightly after he removes the tube. Then, he'll dress the insertion site as described above.

Thoracentesis

To remove accumulated fluid or air from the patient's pleural cavity, the doctor may do a thoracentesis.

To do so, he'll need assistance. Can you give it? On these pages, you'll learn how to help before, during, and after the procedure. In addition, you'll find instructions on using equipment, evaluating your patient's pleural fluid, and preparing any biopsy specimens the doctor may remove for the lab.

When thoracentesis is indicated

Do areas of your patient's chest sound dull when you're percussing them? Are his breath sounds diminished when you listen through a stethoscope? Does X-ray examination reveal a line density in his pleural space? If so, he may have a pleural effusion, which is an accumulation of fluid in his pleural space.

Possible causes include lung infection, pleurisy, cardiovascular or kidney disease, or malignant tumor. Pleural effusion may also be caused by an inflammation in another area of the patient's body. For example, in acute pancreatitis, fluid may migrate from the patient's abdomen to his thoracic cavity.

If the doctor suspects pleural effusion, he may perform a thoracentesis to relieve the patient's symptoms of pain and dyspnea, and to determine what's causing the effusion. To aid in diagnosis, he'll obtain specimens of fluid and possibly biopsied pleural tissue for laboratory analysis.

Assembling the equipment

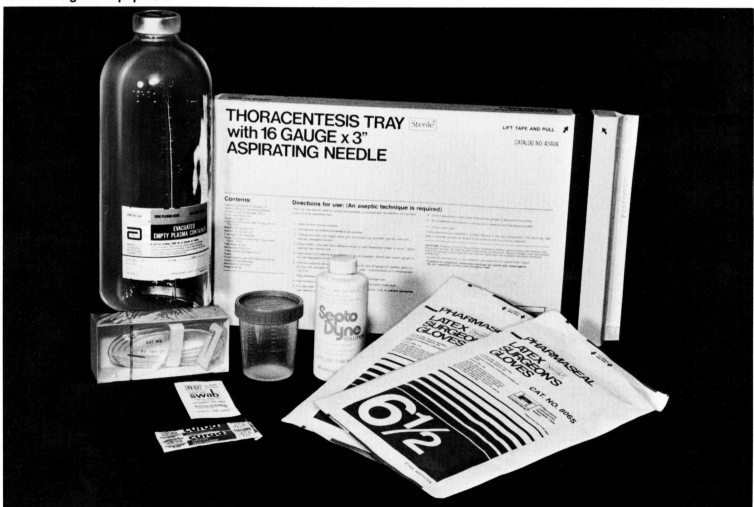

Has the doctor decided that your patient needs a thoracentesis? If so, you'll need to assemble the equipment required to do the procedure, as shown in this photo: thoracentesis tray, sterile gloves, skin disinfectant, local anesthetic, sterile vacuum bottle and tubes, bandage strip, sterile container with formalin (for biopsy).

Also, ask the doctor which type of biopsy needle he'll need (if any), and obtain it from central supply. *Nursing tip:* To help get fluid and biopsy specimens to the lab promptly, prepare specimen labels and requisition slips ahead of time. Learn how to care for the specimens properly on page 154.

Thoracentesis

Thoracentesis: How to position your patient

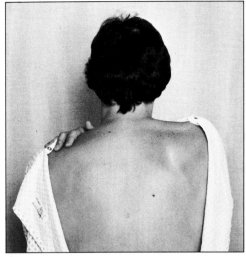

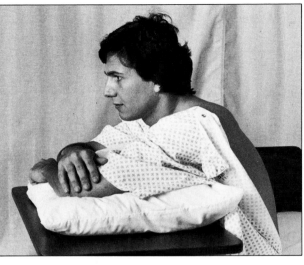

2 Some doctors prefer the patient positioned this way for the procedure. Besides being more comfortable for the patient than sitting straight, this position gives him additional support and keeps his arms out of the way. *Caution:* If you use this position, be sure to lock the bedside table's wheels to keep it from rolling.

1 *You've assembled all the necessary equipment. The doctor has explained the procedure to the patient and has obtained his written consent. Your next step's to position him properly. Depending on your doctor's preference, use one of the positions shown here. As you work, do your best to help your patient relax. Answer any additional questions he may have about the procedure.*

For the position shown above, instruct your patient to sit on the edge of the bed with his feet supported. Find out which side of the patient's chest the doctor plans to tap. Then, tell the patient to place his hand on the opposite shoulder to keep his arm out of the way. As you can see in this photo, the doctor's selected the patient's right side for the procedure.

3 If your patient has trouble sitting up, the doctor may ask you to position him lying down, as shown here. Make sure the patient lies on his unaffected side, close to the edge of the bed. Ask him to place his arm like the patient's doing in this photo. This will help separate his ribs at the puncture site.

Thoracentesis: Assisting with the procedure

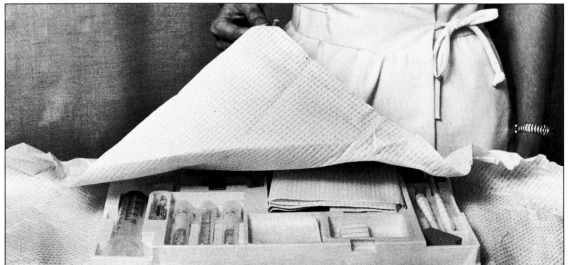

1 *Let's assume that you've already positioned your patient, and the doctor has determined the needle insertion site. Here's what to do next:*

Start with a disposable thoracentesis unit, if your hospital uses them. Now, open the box containing the thoracentesis tray and unwrap the sterile drape, taking care not to contaminate its inner surface.

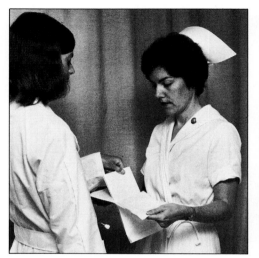

2 Next, open the packet that contains the sterile gloves. The doctor will then remove the inner envelope and slip on the gloves. From this point until the procedure is over, only the doctor will touch the patient. Depending on the doctor's preference, have a hemostat available. She may wish to attach it to the needle to keep it from accidentally penetrating too deeply and injuring the patient's lung.

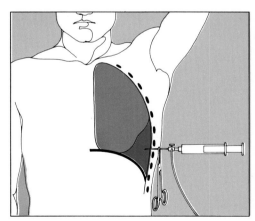

3 To perform the thoracentesis, the doctor first cleans the skin around the puncture site with povidone-iodine solution. Then, she drapes the area with sterile towels. Using a 5 ml syringe, she injects the site with a local anesthetic such as lidocaine, creating a skin wheal. With a larger needle, she then infiltrates the intercostal muscles with anesthetic. After this, she switches to a 50 ml syringe with a 3″ long large-bore (16G) needle and a three-way stopcock.

Warn your patient that he may feel a sudden twinge of pain as the needle penetrates deeper. Remind him not to move or cough while the needle's in his chest wall.

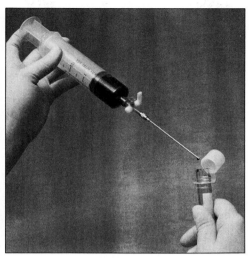

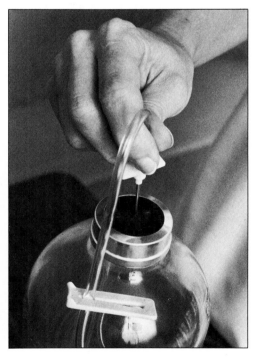

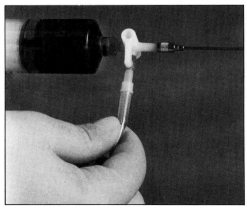

4 As soon as the needle has pierced the outer pleura, the doctor can aspirate fluid into the syringe. If she wants laboratory studies done, she'll fill the syringe, rotate the stopcock, and eject the fluid into three different sterile tubes for bacteriology, chemistry, and histology tests. Send these fluid samples to the lab immediately, along with any biopsy specimens. (For detailed instructions on how to care for a lab specimen, see page 154.)

Throughout the procedure, watch your patient closely; assess his skin color, pulse, and breathing pattern. *Caution:* Sudden change of pressure on the thoracic organs may cause fainting.

5 If the patient has a large effusion, the doctor may want a vacuum bottle for drainage. How can you help? Remove the vacuum bottle's metal lid, exposing the rubber stopper. Pick up the connecting tube and uncap the needle. To prevent vacuum loss, clamp the tube shut with its own sliding clamp, as shown in this photo. Then, insert the needle through the X in the bottle's stopper.

6 Now, connect the other end of the tube to the syringe's stopcock port and open the sliding clamp. Stand by as the doctor opens the syringe port. This will allow pleural fluid to drain through the tube into the vacuum bottle.

When drainage is complete, the doctor will withdraw the needle and place a dry sterile dressing over the puncture site. To help evaluate the procedure's effectiveness and to check for possible pneumothorax, she'll probably request an immediate portable X-ray examination.

Thoracentesis

After thoracentesis: How to care for the patient

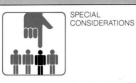

SPECIAL
CONSIDERATIONS

Caring for your patient. After the procedure's over, reassure your patient and allow him to rest for a few hours. Watch him closely for possible complications, for example, pneumothorax or lung tissue damage. To check for lung tissue damage, observe your patient's sputum for traces of blood. To watch for pneumothorax, check his signs at least once every 30 minutes.

Signs and symptoms of pneumothorax include increased respiratory rate, increased pulse rate, blood pressure changes, skin color changes (cyanosis or pallor), asymmetric chest expansion, dyspnea, chest pain, and diminished or absent breath sounds on the affected side. If you strongly suspect a pneumothorax, notify the doctor immediately and begin giving the patient oxygen. The doctor'll probably order a portable chest X-ray exam. If the results confirm a pneumothorax, be prepared to help insert chest tubes, as explained on page 138.

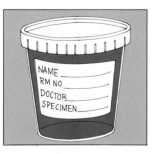

Charting. Document the procedure, including the doctor's name, time when the procedure began and ended, and color and amount of pleural fluid obtained. Indicate whether you sent specimens to the lab, as well as which studies the doctor ordered. Also indicate how well your patient tolerated the procedure; record his vital signs both before and after thoracentesis. Finally, be sure to include date, time, and your signature.

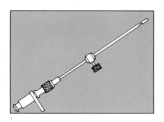

Caring for laboratory specimens. Send specimen containers to the lab promptly. Make sure they're correctly labeled with your patient's name, room number, and doctor's name. Include properly filled-out requisition slips. Remember, some tests require warm specimens; others may require biopsy specimens in saline solution or formalin. To make sure specimens are usable when they get to the lab, check first with laboratory personnel for instructions.

NAME
RM NO
DOCTOR
SPECIMEN

Caring for equipment. Dispose of needles and syringes correctly. Discard all nonreusable materials. Did the doctor use a biopsy needle? Carefully clean it and return it intact to central supply for sterilization and recycling.

Examining pleural fluid

What does the appearance of your patient's pleural fluid tell you about his condition? Is it clear? Bloody? While the appearance can give you a clue—it isn't decisive. Other studies done in the laboratory may help determine your patient's diagnosis. Check the following chart for guidelines on appearance:

Appearance of pleural fluid	Possible cause
Light, straw-colored	• Normal
Purulent	• Empyema
Blood-tinged	• Hemothorax • TB • Pulmonary infarction • Neoplastic disease • Accidental tissue damage from thoracentesis.
Milky (chylothorax)	• Invasion of thoracic duct by a tumor, or an inflammatory process • Traumatic rupture of thoracic duct • Cellular debris or cholesterol crystals.

Test	Interpretation
Gram's stain culture and sensitivity	• If positive, it may mean the early stages of bacterial infection. *Remember:* In the later stages of bacterial infection, the fluid may look grossly purulent with a positive Gram's stain, yet cultures may be negative from antibiotic therapy.
Acid-fast stain and culture	• If positive, it may mean TB.
Red blood cells	• If count is about 10,000 per cu mm and the specimen's pink or light red in color, it may indicate tissue damage. • If count is above 100,000 per cu mm and the specimen's grossly bloody, it suggests intrapleural malignancy, pulmonary infarction, TB, or closed chest trauma. If a hemothorax is present, the hematocrit of the pleural fluid will be similar to the hematocrit of capillary blood.
Leukocytes	• If count is above 1,000 per cu mm or above 50% neutrophils, it may indicate septic or nonseptic inflammation.
Lymphocytes	• If count is over 50%, it may mean TB, or lymphoma or other form of cancer.
Blood clots	• If present, it may mean neoplasm, TB, or infection.
Specific gravity	• If measurement is above 1.016, it may mean neoplasm, TB, or infection. • If measurement is less than 1.104, it may mean congestive heart failure.
Total protein	• If measurement is above 3, it may mean congestive heart failure. • If measurement is less than 3, it suggests neoplasm, TB, or infection.
Lactic dehydrogenase (LDH)	• Measurement increased in cancer. • Measurement decreased in heart failure.
Glucose	• If less than serum glucose, it may mean cancer or a bacterial infection such as TB, or nonseptic inflammation.
Sediment	• If present, it may be cancerous cells, cellular debris, or cholesterol crystals.
Biopsy	• May reveal a tumor.

Suggested further reading

Bendixen, Henrik H., et al. RESPIRATORY CARE. St. Louis: C. V. Mosby Company, 1965.

Burton, George G., et al. RESPIRATORY CARE: A GUIDE TO CLINICAL PRACTICE. Philadelphia: J. B. Lippincott Company, 1977.

Bushnell, Sharon S. RESPIRATORY INTENSIVE CARE NURSING. From Beth Israel Hospital. Boston: Little, Brown and Company, 1973.

Cherniack, Rueben M., et al. RESPIRATION IN HEALTH AND DISEASE. Philadelphia: W. B. Saunders Company, 1972.

Degowin, Elmer, and Richard L. Degowin. BEDSIDE DIAGNOSTIC EXAMINATION. New York: Macmillan Publishing Company, Inc., 1976.

Dripps, Robert, et al. INTRODUCTION TO ANESTHESIA: THE PRINCIPLES OF SAFE PRACTICE. Philadelphia: W. B. Saunders Company, 1977.

Egan, Donald F. FUNDAMENTALS OF RESPIRATORY THERAPY. St. Louis: C. V. Mosby Company, 1977.

Glover, Dennis W., and Margaret M. Glover. RESPIRATORY THERAPY: BASICS FOR NURSING AND THE ALLIED HEALTH PROFESSIONS. St. Louis: C. V. Mosby Company, 1978.

Guyton, Arthur C. TEXTBOOK OF MEDICAL PHYSIOLOGY. Philadelphia: W. B. Saunders Company, 1976.

Judge, Richard D., and George D. Zuidema, eds. METHODS OF CLINICAL EXAMINATION: A PHYSIOLOGIC APPROACH. Boston: Little, Brown and Company, 1974.

Lillington, Glen A. DIAGNOSTIC APPROACH TO CHEST DISEASES. Baltimore: Williams and Wilkins Company, 1977.

Malasanos, Lois, et al. HEALTH ASSESSMENT. St. Louis: C. V. Mosby Company, 1977.

Meltzer, L. E., et al. CONCEPTS AND PRACTICES OF INTENSIVE CARE FOR NURSE SPECIALISTS. Bowie, Md.: Charles Press Publishers, 1976.

Middleton, Elliott, and Charles E. Reed. ALLERGY: PRINCIPLES AND PRACTICE. St. Louis: C. V. Mosby Company, 1978.

Netter, Frank, illus. RESPIRATORY SYSTEM, VOLUME 7. (Medical Illustrations) Summit, N.J.: CIBA Pharmaceuticals, 1979.

Norris, Walter, and Donald Campbell. A NURSES' GUIDE TO ANAESTHETICS, RESUSCITATION AND INTENSIVE CARE. New York: Churchill Livingstone, 1976.

Nursing79 Books. NURSE'S GUIDE TO DRUGS. Horsham, Pa.: Intermed Communications, Inc., 1979.

Sagel, Stuart S. SPECIAL PROCEDURES IN CHEST RADIOLOGY. Philadelphia: W. B. Saunders Company, 1976.

Sana, Josephine, and Richard Judge, eds. PHYSICAL APPRAISAL METHODS IN NURSING PRACTICE. Boston: Little, Brown and Company, 1975.

Shapiro, Barry A., et al. CLINICAL APPLICATION OF RESPIRATORY CARE. Chicago: Yearbook Medical Publishers, 1975.

Thompson, Thomas T. PRIMER OF CLINICAL RADIOLOGY. Boston: Little, Brown and Company, 1973.

Wade, Jacqueline F. RESPIRATORY NURSING CARE: PHYSIOLOGY AND TECHNIQUE, 2nd ed. St. Louis: C. V. Mosby Company, 1977.

Acknowledgements

We'd like to thank the following people
and companies for their help with this PHOTOBOOK:

A-PRN, Inc. (Acute Patient Rental Needs), Mount Laurel, N. J.;
Lee Weiler, Vice President

J. H. Emerson Company, Cambridge, Mass.; Will Emerson

Healthco, Inc., Reading, Pa.; Al Szymborski, CMR

Lekites Oxygen Therapy Company, North Wales, Pa.

Narco Air-Shields, Division of NARCO Scientific, Hatboro, Pa.

Ohio Medical Products, Division of AIRCO, Inc., Madison, Wis.

Puritan-Bennett Corporation, Bellmawr, N. J.; Joe Fleming

The Silver Dry Goods Company, Inc., Philadelphia, Pa.

Also the staffs of:

Delaware Valley Medical Center, Bristol, Pa.

Doylestown Hospital, Doylestown, Pa.

Germantown Hospital, Philadelphia, Pa.

Temple University Hospital, Philadelphia, Pa.

Winter Park Memorial Hospital, Winter Park, Fla.

Index

Index

Index